HEALING
POWER
OF
YOU

HEALING
POWER
OF
YOU

A GUIDE TO WELLNESS AND HEALING

DR. KEITH POORBAUGH

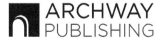
ARCHWAY
PUBLISHING

Archway Publishing books may be ordered through booksellers or by contacting:

Archway Publishing
1663 Liberty Drive
Bloomington, IN 47403
www.archwaypublishing.com
1 (888) 242-5904

ISBN: 978-1-4808-9011-4 (sc)
ISBN: 978-1-4808-9009-1 (hc)
ISBN: 978-1-4808-9010-7 (e)

Library of Congress Control Number: 2020910794

Print information available on the last page.

Archway Publishing rev. date: 6/23/2020

For those who struggle with pain, may your path lead towards a better life.
—KEITH POORBAUGH

CONTENTS

FOREWORD

Never before has there been a time in such need of truth and clarity for understanding and managing pain. Perhaps some people lack the courage to speak what they experience as truth for fear of disturbing the illusion. For more than 25 years as a Doctor of Physical Therapy, Keith Poorbaugh has learned the truth about the healing power of movement through extensive study and the plight of his clients. Imagine if you will, a person struggling with immeasurable chronic pain, suffering beyond the realm of reason, looking for sanctuary in a medical system that has promised an opportunity to be rid of such afflictions. Yet the reality is traditional medical care continues to fail those suffering with musculo-skeletal pain. Again and again.

It is not the failure of the system, it's the illusion of a fix. The lens that the medical system peers through is only focused on pathology and disease. Thankfully, they have the most advanced tools and talented experts to combat illness, injury, and infection. However, there is one blind spot that continues to plague healthcare. Pain associated with movement does not fit neatly into the medical model of disease. When it comes to musculoskeletal pain, humans have the capacity to heal themselves. The issue at hand is that we must begin to respect healing as the primary remedy for pain. Since healthcare can't make the transition to this reality, the power of healing is left to the individual.

In the book, *"Healing Power of You"*, Dr. Poorbaugh guides us along the path of healing by explaining how the musculoskeletal chain truly functions and outlining how we can create a healing environment using proven methods and tools to trigger the healing power that exists in each of us. Dr. Poorbaugh shares with the reader his insights into a very complicated process yet makes it easy to understand and applicable for anyone suffering with musculoskeletal pain. His relentless persistence to create a relevant model that is scientifically based and empirically sound is a testament to his endless pursuit of clinical expertise and practical experiences. This book sheds light on the campaign of misinformation and broken promises that leaves so many frustrated with the traditional medical management of musculoskeletal pain. Dr. Poorbaugh gives the reader the opportunity to learn about the balance of structure and function within the musculoskeletal chain and its amazing healing power.

I expect your life will be changed by reading this book. Not for mere sake of learning novel movements or balanced exercises but the knowledge which yields healing power. You will have a new appreciation of the dangers of seeking the medical fix and understand why healthcare is not well-suited for resolving pain. You will understand that your pain is real, it presents itself as an opportunity, it is more a gift than an obstacle. You will regain hope and confidence in a path towards pain relief. Throughout this book you will recount your own memories of pain and relate to the stories of clients struggling with pain relief. Dr. Poorbaugh has clearly defined musculoskeletal pain, how to manage it naturally with the power of movement and how we can take advantage of the opportunity that pain provides. The reality is that the human body wants and needs movement. It is designed to move and willing to heal. Much like a race car is designed to drive fast, we must provide the human architecture with the environment it deserves. The movement system is the most brilliant organic machine the world's greatest minds have ever tried to understand. We are meant to move, often and variably. Let that happen and you will heal.

I believe that you will discover the purpose of pain and learn the path towards healing naturally after reading "Healing Power of You." I believe that you will have the courage to reach out beyond the traditional model of healthcare and seek the intervention and guidance you need for your wellness and healing.

As I write this foreword, we are struggling to survive a global pandemic known as the Coronavirus or Covid-19 Virus. The entire world is experiencing, for some of us the first time, the need to unite against an invader that is invisible and attacks the weakest among us. The elderly and people who are immune system compromised are most vulnerable to this novel virus. We need our healthcare system to stand ready and do what it does best, fight pathology and disease. We are fortunate to have the help of talented medical experts and infection specialists to eradicate this invader. We need the experts to lead that fight. Experts who are trained in the art of dealing with this disease.

While most musculoskeletal dysfunctions and injuries are not life threatening, they should not be looked at with the same lens as the virus or any other disease. We need real experts, the movement experts and physical therapy professionals to be on the front lines of the sedentary behavior pandemic. These movement professionals spend their entire careers dedicated to the pursuit of understanding function of the human body through the lens of movement. The scientific truths that govern physiology are rooted in movement. Physiology is our response to stress and environment. We need experts who help give patients the tools to eliminate their pain through a natural and proven process; Dr. Poorbaugh is one of those experts. He has the courage to stand up for what is true and confront the pain epidemic head on. He has proven to be one of the bright minds to lead us to fully understand the power of pain and the miracle of self-healing. He could not be any bolder in stating the reality, movement is medicine and it is a powerful remedy for pain. My hope is that healthcare will transform to allow physicians around the world to prescribe movement and activity as medicine.

I have been fortunate to have spent time with Dr. Poorbaugh and his colleagues at his clinic. I have enjoyed time with him and his family at his retreat in Willow, Alaska. We have shared movement experiences, nature, healing practices, and personal stories of overcoming adversity and hardship. Yet the one single, common thread we share is the passion for coaching others on their quest for optimal health. We have a desire to continue to learn and to solve the world's human movement problems. Keith has been a military soldier and fighting for others is what he does. I am fortunate to call Keith my friend. His family has welcomed me with open arms, and his colleagues have treated me as one of their own.

I hope that you feel the same way as I did when you read this book. It is a glimpse of the brilliance of this man, his lifelong passion for healing and a glimmer into his authentic spirit.

As pain is a gift, so too is *"Healing Power of You"*.

John Sinclair, BPE, CSCS, CPT, MES, CAFS
Co-Founder, Author and Chief Movement Engineer
Seven Movements
www.sevenmovements.com

Founder
Authentic Health Coaching
www.authentichealthcoaching.com

INTRODUCTION

When you hurt, you want answers. What caused the pain? What can you do to get better? How long will it take? The sad reality is that many people struggling with musculoskeletal pain fail to find consistent or useful answers. This is the challenge we all face. A reliable solution to pain is not readily available. If you search the web, the choices are nearly endless. Often you could end up with more questions than answers, wondering whether your pain is due to serious damage or some illusive syndrome. Of course, there are plenty of recommendations online touting pain relief. Yet most of the remedies lack any relevance and could actually make symptoms worsen. If you seek medical care, there's a good chance you will be offered the standard fix of imaging, drugs, and procedures. Although it's important to consult with a trusted medical provider to rule out any serious disorders when faced with persistent or severe pain, too often the emphasis of medical care is focused on fixing the pain rather than addressing the problem. Unfortunately, the solution to musculoskeletal pain can rarely be found on the web or in the medical office. It's no wonder so many Americans are struggling with chronic musculoskeletal pain. According to a study by the Committee on Advancing Pain Research, common chronic pain conditions affect approximately one hundred million adults in the United States. At a cost of nearly $800 billion annually (Yelin 2016) for medical management, it's time to end the mystery for pain relief. Now more than ever, it's time to discover a safe and effective path to pain relief.

Want to live a life with less pain? This is your chance to learn how to heal and be well. There is no need to restrict activity to avoid pain. Instead, it's time to heal so you can return to activity. If you are willing to focus on movement, instead of pain, then you're ready to restore wellness and tap into the healing potential of the musculoskeletal system. Like most people, I'm sure you're tired of the status quo treatments for pain. No pill or procedure can match the healing potential stored within each link of the musculoskeletal chain. If you are ready to start moving to heal, this book is a must-read to unlock the hidden mysteries behind why we hurt and how to heal. If you are serious about accepting the challenge to defend your body from the damage of today's convenience society, then this book will help you build and defend wellness. If you are a caregiver who is tired of the excessive medicalization of musculoskeletal pain, this book will guide you to a deeper understanding of the path to healing.

Every well human moves to heal. Rediscover the true nature of tissue healing to foster natural pain relief from musculoskeletal conditions. I am always thrilled to share healing stories with my clients. Still, for so many, it's the first time they have had the opportunity to consider that their pain is not a permanent or terminal condition. Too often they are misled by threatening tissue changes shown on imaging (x-ray or MRI). With such evidence of structural damage, it's easy for patients to be convinced that there's only one real solution for the pain. The stark images of tissue degeneration make a good case for the path toward the medical fix. My passion is showing clients a different path. Often, I am the first clinician to explain how pain does not equal tissue damage. Yes, the imaging may show changes in tissue structure, but this can be overcome with changes in tissue function. It's often difficult for a person in pain to accept such a novel idea—the idea that pain can heal instead of being fixed.

I'm not a likely spokesperson for healing. I take great pride in being the adopted son of hardworking parents, neither of whom went to college or even finished high school. In fact, my parents first met while working at a wheat-threshing camp. My father worked the fields, and my mother was a camp cook. Not surprisingly, once they moved from the fields to the city, their expectations were tempered by their lack of skill and education. Yet they relied upon their strong work ethic and faith to provide for their family. Somehow, I managed to put these attributes to work in my life, although not as gracefully as my parents. Still, I managed to make the unusual transition from an airman in the US Air Force to a commissioned officer in the US Army, just hoping to gain some respect. Later, I graduated from one of the most prestigious schools in health science at Mayo Clinic, just hoping to prove that I was smart. Now, I am a physical therapist and hopeful healer, just to test my faith. So why have I written a book on healing? Not because I want respect, because it can only be earned. Not because I'm smart, because it just aren't true. Whether it's my faith in God or passion for healing, the reality is that I care deeply for those who struggle with pain. I refuse to accept the notion that some people are destined to live in pain. Yes, there is definitely something missing in the standard medical approach to pain. It seems that we have become so fascinated by the promise of a pain fix that we have ignored the healing potential of the musculoskeletal system. Yet we have all experienced the reality that pain heals. Convincing clients of the reality that pain heals can be quite challenging. Hopefully I will give you every reason to choose healing as the best option for musculoskeletal pain.

In this book, I will share some insights from my personal and clinical experience to help explain the cause of musculoskeletal pain. Even better, I will offer a rationale based upon recent scientific evidence that demonstrates the danger of choosing a fix instead of the path toward wellness and healing. This book relies on countless hours of client interviews to get the entire story behind musculoskeletal pain while implementing real changes—changes that are capable of restoring tissue health to achieve optimal function and pain relief. This is your opportunity to explore what we know to date on the mystery of healing pain. Science is always changing, but one thing remains true and constant: the musculoskeletal system is designed to heal.

Healing is powered by movement, which makes movement fundamental to our survival. Stasis is not our friend. Less activity and static postures are the hallmarks of pain. How we move to survive the toils and struggles of our daily life is directly related to our ability to heal. Some struggles build our healing potential, while others may weaken it. Mother's old adage, *if it doesn't kill you, it makes you stronger*, may hold some truth. We suffer pain in many ways, whether emotional, social, or physical. Our struggle to restore movement and regain function is directly related to our survival. It's tough to keep a good healer down. Healing can become a habit and a lifestyle. Yet it is not a guarantee. The modern lifestyle of convenience and comfort are not well suited for strengthening our struggle to survive. Yet some things never change. The struggles we face in life are immensely critical to help our nervous system build pathways and patterns that enhance healing potential. Every physical challenge we face creates an opportunity to move and heal. Too often, the opportunity to heal is supplanted by the promise of a quick fix.

There is value in the struggle to heal yourself. Your healing potential becomes stronger every time you turn a painful challenge into a healing opportunity.

Healing is the most critical function of every living cell. We simply can't live or exist without the ability to self-repair. Yet healing does not only occur on a cellular level. We also have the potential to heal on a systemic level. Healing the musculoskeletal system requires some preparation to restore function and establish an optimal level of wellness. Luckily for us, perfection is not required to achieve pain relief. My favorite explanation for healing musculoskeletal pain is not exactly flashy. "I will be your guide along a path of change to improve wellness and restore healing potential so you can return to your previously dysfunctional self." The point is that none of us are perfect. Even prior to pain, our musculoskeletal system was challenged by impaired wellness and imbalances in tissue structure and function. Pain simply announces that the challenge requires some changes—changes in wellness to improve health and changes in movement to improve healing potential.

The human movement system requires a strong mind and healthy body; essentially, quality of life is dependent upon brains and brawn. Achieving the ultimate balance is not necessary, but it's our challenge to build fitness of mind and body to ward off the dangers in life. This fitness comes in the form of wellness and healing potential. Whether it's simple transitions from the floor or lifting a heavy load, nothing is for nothing. Every movement and task creates tissue load that must be absorbed by the musculoskeletal system. The load ability of tissue can be defined by posture and movement. Accepting a load or applying load in a certain position will determine the level of effort necessary to resist or support the load. While movement requires tensile loads throughout the musculoskeletal chain. The external loads our musculoskeletal chain must react to include the ground reaction forces and applied loads during an activity or task. Even more important is the internal loading which occurs within each link and path of the musculoskeletal chain as it generates tension to sustain purposeful movement and compression to maintain joint stability. The combined loads of reaction and generation sets the stage for tissue loading. Tissue loading is dependent upon posture and movement as each segment in the skeletal chain and myofascial paths must respond to forces in nature and within the body. How our tissue responds to loading is variable and remains in a constant flux, but it's immensely dependent upon wellness. How well we care for our body and mind is the foundation for accessing healing potential. The musculoskeletal system is reliant upon an optimal flow of blood and nerve conduction. Keeping our body well rested, active, mentally fit, and fueled by a healthy diet is the best defense against musculoskeletal pain and disease.

The soft tissue supports and moves the hard tissue through a balance of myofascial tension and joint compression. Tension requires freedom of movement and friction-free gliding between multiple layers of muscles and fascia. Soft tissue is aligned to create pathways of tension which are highly dependent on movement for hydration and nutrition. Compression is the pinnacle of stability for the skeletal joints which also maintains a hydrophilic nature due to the presence of cartilage and ligaments. Together the musculoskeletal system is designed for shock absorption and movement with a singular purpose: balance tension to withstand tissue loading. Like the mast and sails on a clipper, our skeletal system would be useless without the myofascial tension that stretches from heel to head. Life is movement. Each segment and link of the musculoskeletal chain is dependent upon movement. Freedom of movement is often taken for granted. Ask anyone suffering painful movement what they wish for most. To move without pain is not only a desire, it's a passion. Pain-free motion allows us to demonstrate the beauty and complexity of movement while achieving the simplest to most difficult tasks—though it does not come without risks.

Pain is not just a possibility; it's a guarantee. Eventually there is a consequence to impaired wellness and limited movement. Whether it's a health stressor or impaired movement, the outcome is tissue overload. Unbeknownst to us, our nervous system utilizes pain to signal the presence of tissue overload. Our response to pain guides the nervous system to alter movement patterns and adapt different muscle strategies to stay on task. The task driven nature of the nervous system keeps our movement system in a relative state of compensation to achieve balance between structure and function. Coordinated activation of muscles and connective tissue are necessary to align joint spaces while creating movement for a given task with minimal effort and energy. These compensatory patterns of movement will either help restore balance to tissue loading or lead to further tissue overload. The outcome is entirely dependent upon the level of wellness and healing potential available. Wellness supports the function of every living cell. If our wellness safe is lacking critical elements or the healing potential is limited, then there's a good chance for pain to persist. Healing potential requires a process of building up and breaking down to restore balance to movement and loading. Pain gives us the motivation to take the necessary steps to build better movement, strength, and stability. Pain is a good reason to break down the old patterns of poor posture and impaired movement that were contributing to tissue overload. We rarely accept change without a reason, and pain is the universal reason for change.

Sooner or later, tissue overload becomes significant to trigger a cycle of pain and inflammation. Pain that limits movement and activity is defined as musculoskeletal pain, while pain that affects systemic bodily functions is known as visceral pain. One is quite irritating and debilitating, while the other is dead serious. Visceral pain and its underlying systemic conditions are not covered in this book. Our focus is solely limited to musculoskeletal pain. Musculoskeletal pain bears all the hallmarks of somatic pain. Traditionally, we associate pain directly with tissue damage. Pain due to significant trauma, such as a twisted ankle during a basketball game or a torn rotator cuff from a FOOSH (falling on outstretched hand), is associated with structural lesions of the movement system. In cases of acute trauma or injury, it is vital to determine exactly what damage has occurred to assist with proper medical management. However, what about the bum knee or aching back that gradually develops overtime? Or the stiff and painful shoulder that starts to limit reaching? Are these conditions still caused by tissue damage? The main problem with the traditional viewpoint of musculoskeletal pain is it fails to recognize the combined role of structure and function within the movement system. Musculoskeletal pain is not determined by structure alone. In the acute setting, stability of structure is the priority. However, in the majority of cases where trauma or injury are not directly related to pain, there's more to the pain equation than just structure. In fact, the movement system is far more reliant upon function to compensate for impairments and deficits within the movement structures.

By the time you complete this book, it should be quite clear that musculoskeletal pain is not solely caused by tissue damage. The human movement system is designed to adapt and overcome imbalances with gradual changes in function despite minor or significant alterations in structure.

But it's a two-way street. Sometimes dysfunction can lead to adaptations in structure, thus creating a weak or degenerated segment. All tissue adapts due to loading and aging, while function readily changes to meet the demands of movement and wellness. If you can change function to better support the movement structure, then pain relief is possible, despite the presence of tissue damage.

Musculoskeletal conditions are the most common causes of pain related to the health and function of the human movement system. Although musculoskeletal conditions are not life-threatening, they can still be harmful. Painful joints and soft tissue dysfunctions tend to be chronic and frequently cause disability (Buchman 2010). According to the World Health Organization, musculoskeletal conditions are the second largest contributor to disability worldwide, with low back pain (LBP) being the single leading cause of disability. Musculoskeletal conditions involve inflammation, irritation, and (or) pain originating from muscles and fascia (myofascial), ligaments, and joints. The primary cause of musculoskeletal dysfunction involves impaired myofascial tension and compensatory movement patterns that lead to an imbalance of tissue loading. Adverse tissue loading can occur at one or more segments of the musculoskeletal chain, causing weak or degenerated segments of the chain to experience tissue overload in the form of either misuse, overuse, or disuse (MOD). Tissue overload at a restricted segment may breach the threshold for tissue alliance and trigger a cycle of pain and inflammation. Once movement becomes painful, the choice is clear: either fear pain and avoid movement or begin the journey for healing. Both are very different paths with the same goal: pain relief.

It's easy to understand how pain forces us to seek a change. No one wants to accept painful movement; therefore, the stakes can be high. Some people take the *grin and bear it* approach as they limp and stagger to reduce loading. I've heard the claims "I live with pain" or "I have a high pain tolerance" only to witness the same person move with compensatory patterns or awkward postures. Ignoring pain is not a reasonable path towards healing. Our nervous system does not ask for permission to adapt to impaired structure or limited function. Ignoring pain only leads to more possibility for tissue overload (MOD) at other sites within the musculoskeletal chain. The *stop and desist* approach is another common response to pain. Our musculoskeletal system is dependent upon variable types of movement to maintain healing potential. Movement powers healing. Limiting movement of tissue simply leads to tissue ischemia (reduced blood flow), which impairs healing. Unfortunately, there's no easy remedy for musculoskeletal pain. Pain is not to be ignored or avoided; instead, it demands change that leads to healing movements and improved wellness.

If musculoskeletal pain is not a sign of tissue damage, then what's the point? No use denying it, pain of this nature must be recognized as an opportunity. Pain is an important notice of dysfunction or imbalance within the musculoskeletal system. Rather than a warning, it's a ping from the nervous system designed to grab our attention and steer us toward an opportunity for change. The tone and volume of the ping is related to prior pain experiences and current perspectives. If you've had serious challenges with recovering from pain, then fear and avoidance may heighten pain intensity and make recovery even more challenging. Or if you doubt your chances for recovery and become anxious about returning to activity, then it can be the start of a self-fulfilling prophecy. Still, neither the pain intensity nor the duration matters, except of course to the pain sufferer. Since musculoskeletal pain is not a sign of tissue damage or danger, there is only one message that demands our attention: it's time to change.

Pain is fuel for change. Pain brings about changes in the movement system ranging from avoidance to confrontation. If a region of the musculoskeletal chain is stiff, weak, or unstable, then the options are limited. The nervous system must adapt to these functional imbalances using whatever is available at the moment within the movement system. In the case of weakness, it will disrupt the balance of tension throughout an entire myofascial loop. This discontinuous tension may cause tissue overload in the form of impaired joint stability or muscular weakness. In the presence of stiffness, our neural drive reduces tension in paths of the myofascial loop by delaying or avoiding activation of tension which may impair shock absorption from nearby segments. Thus stiff segments in the chain are predisposed to tissue overload from a lack of strength and inadequate tissue nutrition. None of these adaptations are perfect solutions, but the nervous system must balance myofascial tension and joint compression to keep the musculoskeletal chain mobile and responsive to loading. Oftentimes, adaptations in function and compensatory movement patterns put the musculoskeletal chain at risk for tissue overload (MOD), which can lead to pain and inflammation.

Pain is the rugged mountain reflected in the calm lake. It makes us consider the value of our actions and purpose of our movement. Fear of movement or avoidance of activity does not promote healing or pain relief. In fact, it could lead to the exact opposite. Limiting participation in work and social life tends to heighten the awareness of pain. Restricting movement only results in poor control of muscle activation and increased risk for tissue overload. Pain should not be ignored or avoided; instead, it should be recognized as an opportunity to protect and defend our musculoskeletal system. Accepting pain as an opportunity opens a PATH toward healing:

1. *Pacing*. Gradual return to activity and movement. Choose familiar activities to begin low-load aerobic challenges. Build your sweat equity.
2. *Awareness*. Practice control of position and effort, better known as postural awareness. Build muscle activation and strength in various postures to enhance awareness.
3. *Timing*. Relearning movement is all about timing and accuracy. Put some skill back into your movements and learn how to play hard without hurting.
4. *Help*. Don't be afraid to get some help and guidance. Some aspects of healing are tough to achieve on your own.

If you are struggling with persistent pain, then it's time to get on the healing path. Become aware of controlled and purposeful movement instead of pain awareness. Pace yourself and return to activity with a zest for skilled movement instead of fear-based avoidance. Seek help to restore mobility, strength, and balance to the entire musculoskeletal chain. This is the most direct route toward natural tissue healing. Healing should be the first consideration for musculoskeletal pain, yet it's all too often ignored.

Medical management has become the standard choice for musculoskeletal pain. It's sleek and sophisticated, but very few people recognize the danger of choosing a medical fix over natural healing. Medical management of musculoskeletal problems has become more business oriented than patient focused. We can't deny the hardships of the health care transition to the business model. Over the last three decades, the pain epidemic has created year-after-year increases in rates of disability for musculoskeletal conditions. The opiate epidemic has led drug overdose to be the most likely cause of accidental death. Sadly, adults in the US are more likely to die from a drug overdose than from a traffic accident or gunshot (CDC).

Many patients are steered toward a medical remedy even though a healing intervention could be a safer and possibly a more effective route. In fact, it reminds me of the forty-two-year-old flight attendant who came to our clinic after surgery. Katie had struggled with severe shoulder pain and stiffness for nearly three years before her most recent surgery—a surgical procedure that was supposed to fix the problem. She was the ideal compliant patient, keeping strict adherence to surgical restrictions and exercise recommendations. Surgery was indicated since she had positive findings on imaging showing a muscle tendon tear and bursitis. Her symptoms warranted consideration for more invasive procedures. Yet she still struggles with the same pain and stiffness that originally led her to surgery.

During our initial consult, Katie recalled a gradual decline of upper extremity function over the course of three years. During that time, it had become nearly impossible to raise her arm above waist height. She still continued to work and even attempted to remain active with family and her favorite recreation, skiing. But as time passed and treatment after treatment failed to yield results, she was convinced that surgery was the only option. Now months after surgery, it seems she is still dealing with the same symptoms. Her shoulder is still extremely stiff, and the pain remains irritable. Is it a failed procedure or simply a flawed process? Unfortunately, since every medical intervention only focused on the painful site, we may never know the answer. For instance, there was no assessment of her musculoskeletal chain to assess whether functional imbalances could have been the barriers to healing. Perhaps a more detailed evaluation would have discovered that she was still struggling from elbow instability after years of playing volleyball in college. Also, it would have determined the presence of hip weakness and back pain which directly limited shoulder stability. The surgery may have repaired the structure, but the functional problems remained. The reality is quite simple: when it comes to musculoskeletal conditions, even surgery can't fix function.

America's healthcare system is ideally suited for treatment and management of trauma, infection, pathology, and surgery (TIPS), but it is not well suited for musculoskeletal pain. All too often, Americans fail to realize the danger of trusting our health care system to resolve musculoskeletal pain with imaging, pills, and procedures. Many people are not aware of the gradual transition of the medical system from evidence-based medicine (EBM) to money-based medicine (MBM). Health care is now health business. Health business has cheated patients with musculoskeletal pain out of their healing potential merely for the sake of higher profit margins. We are bearing witness to a system meltdown where the true intent of the health care model is being exposed by the headlines of rampant addiction to prescription opiates, false advertisements by corporations, and endless stories of patients suffering disability and disappointment.

There is no safe and effective fix for musculoskeletal pain. It's an illusion created through an endless surge of ad campaigns and direct marketing to consumers and medical providers. Just consider the recent trends for medical marketing in the US. From 1997 through 2016, medical marketing expanded substantially, and spending increased from $17.7 to $29.9 billion, with direct-to-consumer advertising for prescription drugs and health services accounting for the most rapid growth and pharmaceutical marketing to health professionals accounting for most promotional spending (Schwartz 2019). Face the truth and ignore the ads; drugs and surgery simply can't replace healing.

Healing is not a place; it's a daily journey. Like every journey, there's more than one path to travel. The path of least resistance requires little consideration for personal wellness and healing potential; it simply requires a willingness to subject your body to expensive and sometimes risky imaging, pills, and procedures. This is the medical fix path where the individual initiates nothing but endures everything. On the other path is wellness and healing. This is the path that is often poorly marked and nearly hidden from view. It requires exploring novel ways to reclaim wellness and restore healing potential with movement. Movement is the key to restoring local tissue nutrition and optimal function. This is the path where the individual initiates everything necessary to restore wellness and activate healing potential within the musculoskeletal chain.

It's important to make a clear distinction between musculoskeletal pain and pain caused by TIPS. Musculoskeletal pain is provoked by a change of posture or movement. It can be dull or sharp in nature, but it's typically relieved by rest or varying posture and movement. TIPS-related pain is poorly patterned and not always directly related to movement. It's necessary to appreciate that pain can be the only indicator of a serious condition or disease. Please seek medical attention if your pain is not related to movement or if pain fails to resolve with rest. Any suspicion or concerns regarding pain possibly related to TIPS should be evaluated by a licensed, qualified, and competent medical provider. Persistent or severe pain should always be evaluated by a medical provider to rule out TIPS.

This book is not intended as a substitute for medical advice. Readers should consult a competent and licensed medical provider in matters relating to health and particularly with respect to any symptoms that may require diagnosis or medical attention. Client stories reflect the author's present recollections of experiences over time. Some names and characteristics have been changed, some events have been compressed, and some dialogue has been recreated.

PAINFUL LIES

It's not by accident or happenstance that Americans have lost faith in the power of healing. It's a predictable response to the coordinated efforts of today's health businesses to reshape the public's image of healing. Over the past few decades, Americans have been misled and cheated out of their healing potential. There's no denying that America has the most advanced medical system in the world. Yet is the medical system the best option for musculoskeletal pain? It's a redundant query, since we have already been conditioned to believe our medical system is able to fix everything, including pain. Perhaps it's time to consider who's really responsible for our wellness and healing.

Unfortunately, it's quite common for people with musculoskeletal pain to believe they simply can't heal. Whether it's because they don't deserve to heal or the condition is too severe to heal, beliefs can have serious consequences. Pain can easily become a heavy emotional toll. Whether it's due to guilt or blame, there are always plenty of opportunities to feel overwhelmed or victimized by the struggle with pain. Yet expecting healing to fail often creates the perfect scenario for accepting the fix. Pain is a burden, and it's just easier to shift responsibility to an apathetic system.

The fix is far removed from the how and why of pain. If the pain increases in severity, then the fix approach assumes the condition involves more damage. This is a common fallacy. Very similar to how a paper cut hurts far more than an open gash. Convincing someone experiencing pain the problem is complex, but the solutions are simple can prove to be a very difficult task. It's more likely that people in severe pain will mistakenly believe only the most powerful pill or invasive procedure can resolve their symptoms. It's easier to believe someone else is responsible for resolving pain, especially if you don't believe you deserve healing or you believe there is no hope for healing. The fact is that healing is available to every well human. There is no risk in hope for healing.

Our identity, beliefs, and habits make Americans primed and willing subjects for the great illusion of a fix. Unfortunately, we have proven ourselves to be fools for the fix. From pioneers to patients, we have conformed to a role of compliance and overreliance. We readily accept prescription drugs to mask pain. Providers and patients yield to insurance dictating and limiting medical care. We rely upon invasive procedures to fix pain while ignoring the risks. We have denied our pioneering spirit as self-healers for the illusion of a fix to musculoskeletal pain. You could argue our belief in the advances and progress of medicine lends credence to the fix. Yet there are few instances where medicine has been proven to fix a disorder, it's more common to have excessive or inadequate treatment with unpredictable costs and risks. All the more reasons why the medical fix for musculoskeletal pain remains poorly defined and mismanaged.

More likely, the allure of a quick fix is supported by our lifestyles. Convenience has supplanted struggle; comfort has replaced necessity. It's a blanket stereotype, but it really sums up the rationale used to justify choosing a fix for pain. No one wants to struggle with pain, but the choice is clear. Healing is not a procedure. Nor can it be prescribed. It's a process that requires time and effort to make real changes in tissue load and nutrition. Unlike the fix, there's no real risk in healing. Perhaps the medical fix would be worth the risks if the final outcome was resolution of pain and restored function, but that's the real kicker: drugs don't cure pain, and surgery doesn't fix function.

The reality is the deck has been stacked against healing for quite some time. There are false fronts on all sides of this struggle to capitalize on the management of musculoskeletal pain. The most fundamental lie is that musculoskeletal conditions must be diagnosed and managed as disease. Jackie Scully, senior research fellow, uses the example of osteoporosis to highlight the problems with labeling musculoskeletal conditions as a disease. In 1994, the World Health Organization (WHO) officially recognized osteoporosis as a disease, which switched it from being an unavoidable part of normal aging to a pathology (Schwartz 2019). Granted, there is no doubt osteoporosis can develop into a debilitating disorder due to severe joint pain and limited mobility, but is it truly a disease? Scully points out that disease status matters because "today's medicine has an unprecedented ability to actually do things, it matters a great deal what we decide to tackle." Perhaps the push to overmedicalize musculoskeletal pain is more related to the fact that insurance and reimbursement are more closely tied to a disease state.

The real damage of using a disease classification for musculoskeletal conditions is the illusion it creates; pain can only be resolved if the problem is fixed. Since it's nearly impossible to identify the functional problems within the movement system related to pain, the fix is directed solely at structural problems identified on imaging. Disease-based management fails to recognize the interdependence of structure and function for balanced support of the musculoskeletal system. There is no value in considering one without the other. The disease approach ignores the true purpose of the musculoskeletal system: movement. Movement is a product of structure and function to achieve a balance of stability and mobility. The presence of some flaw or defect on imaging fails to isolate the true source of pain. Imaging as the sole source of diagnosis is useless for musculoskeletal pain, since the pain is often far removed from the problem. The prescription of disease-based treatment is like using a sledgehammer to tap in a tack. Musculoskeletal pain is not a sign of tissue damage. It is an indication of tissue overload or lack of tissue nutrition, which often only requires a change in wellness and movement to access healing potential.

Musculoskeletal conditions involve normal tissue that is simply inflamed, irritated, or ischemic. A disease approach prefers to isolate pain as being the problem and focuses all attention on the painful site. This approach fails to recognize the real problem is the functional imbalance that caused or led to the structure becoming painful. A disease-based approach to pain casts musculoskeletal dysfunctions into an overtasked medical system geared toward comprehensive, bordering on excessive, disease approaches. Treating musculoskeletal pain as a disease leads to these big three empty promises:

1. Useless and costly imaging to identify structural causes of pain
2. Risky and addictive drugs to eliminate pain

3. Expensive and invasive surgical procedures to correct structural problems

Empty promises form the basis for the overmedicalization of musculoskeletal pain. Perhaps a more relevant example for misclassification of musculoskeletal dysfunctions is the recognition of LBP as a primary disease. The disease label brings with it the full weight of the medical system. Practitioners use every means at their disposal to diagnose and manage the disease until it is cured or fixed. Insurers only authorize treatment for conditions that are properly coded for disease and impairment. Pharmaceuticals use the opportunity to market endless variations of new and existing drugs to cure musculoskeletal disease. If we accept LBP as a disease, the individual and societal burden of disability and dependence will continue to increase, regardless of medical advances. With this disease-based strategy, the medical system has tackled nearly every musculoskeletal condition, thus leading America to have the highest rate of imaging, drug prescriptions, and surgery merely for the sake of abating musculoskeletal pain.

Of course, it's important to rule out any serious pathology that could mimic musculoskeletal pain. Yet the medical narrative and examination have taken a back seat to the advanced technology of modern imaging. Imaging has become the critical factor in determining care and justifying insurance coverage. From 2000 to 2008, there was a 60 percent increase of imaging for musculoskeletal conditions (Rao 2011). Virtually all imaging of musculoskeletal conditions focused on structural findings, which tells us very little in regard to functional imbalances. Most images are taken in an unloaded position, so the true effects of loading are not functional. It's rare for any imaging to include any comparative images of the opposite side or segments adjacent to the pain. Reasons such as these exclude function from the examination process and lead to high rates of false positives and excessive medical treatment. The positive findings of structural damage are often physiological tissue changes (age dependent and completely natural), which occur regardless of pain. Consider this study that shows the imaging findings for asymptomatic (without pain) adults (Brinjikji 2015).

imaging findings in asymptomatic patients[a]

Imaging Finding	Age (yr)						
	20	30	40	50	60	70	80
Disk degeneration	37%	52%	68%	80%	88%	93%	96%
Disk signal loss	17%	33%	54%	73%	86%	94%	97%
Disk height loss	24%	34%	45%	56%	67%	76%	84%
Disk bulge	30%	40%	50%	60%	69%	77%	84%
Disk protrusion	29%	31%	33%	36%	38%	40%	43%
Annular fissure	19%	20%	22%	23%	25%	27%	29%
Facet degeneration	4%	9%	18%	32%	50%	69%	83%
Spondylolisthesis	3%	5%	8%	14%	23%	35%	50%

[a] Prevalence rates estimated with a generalized linear mixed-effects model for the age-specific prevalence estimate (binomial outcome) clustering on study and adjusting for the midpoint of each reported age interval of the study.

Imaging findings of degeneration are common in asymptomatic adults.

Beyond false positives, most degenerative changes shown with imaging are the simple wear and tear of tissue related to stress from our daily lives. Sadly, all living tissue is on the clock—meaning it's destined to tear, degrade, and show signs of stress from tissue loading. Loading causes tissue to adapt and deform. Since the nineteenth century, our understanding of the effects of loading on skeletal bones has evolved from a simple appreciation to a complex question. In 1892, Julius Wolff, a German anatomist and surgeon, recognized that mechanical loads affect bone architecture. Wolff's law was the fundamental principle of how mechanical forces cause living tissue to adapt and mature. For more than a century, we have learned to appreciate that loading is essential for structural stability. It's why every parent is anxious for the day their toddler takes their first step. Intuitively, we all realize the benefits of loading. Even the early researchers appreciated that muscles are the primary structure responsible for loading the skeletal system (Frost 2004). But the effects of loading on pain and function are less evident.

We have moved far beyond Wolff's law in our understanding of how bone loading triggers other systems to respond to sustain tissue health. Yet we continue to omit the purpose of loading within other components of the musculoskeletal system. Optimal loading supports local blood flow and metabolism of muscle and fascia to foster increased strength and resilience. Every fiber and fascicle of the muscles and fascia are dependent upon loading for tissue mobility and nutrition. Improper loading can lead to restrictions in gliding of muscles and fascia along entire pathways, creating an imbalance of tension. These restrictions are represented as impaired or delayed muscle activation and altered movement patterns, which lead to segmental weakness, instability, or stiffness (WIS). As the loads are shifted to other segments within the chain, there is increased potential for tissue overload (MOD), which deprives tissue of local nutrition. Tissue overload may accelerate degenerative changes and trigger a cycle of pain and inflammation.

Most signs of tissue overload identified on imaging require years, likely decades, to develop. If these are long-standing tissue changes that existed well before the onset of pain, how is it possible that fixing the problem on imaging will fix the pain? The painful region is simply experiencing tissue overload due to a functional imbalance somewhere else in the musculoskeletal chain. Imaging is only useful to confirm what we already suspect based upon the detailed history and physical examination. In the case of musculoskeletal pain, imaging is a useful tool to rule out

TIPS. However, imaging fails miserably at determining the true cause of musculoskeletal pain. Yet we continue to see imaging as the cornerstone of the medical fix.

The illusion of a fix for musculoskeletal pain has been sold to the American public for decades as drugs and surgery have become the mainstay of the health care model. Patients are rarely warned about the risks of addiction or disability. Little mention is made of the potential pitfalls that occur as a result of trying to fix the structural problem. Patients are often shown the culprit on imaging and convinced that drugs and surgery are the only option. There are many classes of drugs that are used to treat musculoskeletal pain, ranging from antiinflammation to stimulants and depressants. Still, none of these prescription drugs are designed to trigger tissue repair or restore function. Frankly, a healing drug does not exist.

Most prescription drugs tend to slow or delay the healing process if not combined with movement and nutrition (Aguirre 2016, Wachholtz 2014). Still, the prescribing habits have followed an upward trend, leading to the current opiate crisis where roughly 42 percent to 71 percent of office visits for pain result in a prescription medication (Ferrell 2006). Regardless of the risk of addiction, Americans are still the greatest consumers of opiates in the world. The US comprises 5 percent of the world population, yet we consume 86 percent of all opiates produced worldwide (Riera 2015). Over the past few decades, more potent and powerful drugs have allowed medicine to more effectively treat disease. This is in large part due to increased understanding of genetics and pathology. These same drugs are often marketed off-label for a host of additional conditions and disorders to ramp up sales margin. Using a disease-based drug to manage a musculoskeletal dysfunction is akin to using poison to ward off the effects of a bee sting.

The typical scheme used to get drugs mainstreamed is all about marketing. Like most new drugs, Lyrica was introduced as a limited-use medication to treat a single disorder, epilepsy. However, with the success of the drug against one disease, it's typical to explore off-label applications with scant evidence supporting diversification. Even though Lyrica was primarily launched as an anticonvulsant, it soon became a standard stock of the American medicine cabinet due to an expansion of its off-label prescriptions. Lyrica has experienced enormous growth primarily in its diversification aimed at the treatment of a wide range of musculoskeletal conditions. For instance, direct-to-consumer marketing has been used to promise relief from sciatica, fibromyalgia, and restless leg syndrome. It's also been prescribed to treat anxiety and neuropathic pain. Most of these claims have been debunked by recent research (Violet 2019).

According to a recent court case, Pfizer engaged in extensive direct-to-consumer advertising campaigns to promote Lyrica for fibromyalgia and diabetic nerve pain indications. In 2016, the company spent a record amount, $24.6 million, to market this drug to the public. Reaching global revenues of $14 billion in Lyrica sales demonstrates the value of aggressive advertising. Of course, the cost of this drug staple quadrupled as usage soared. With nearly a million Medicare recipients on prescription Lyrica, the costs in Medicare spending was $2.1 billion in 2016. Pfizer wasn't the only drug company spreading lies during public marketing campaigns. Even trusted companies like Johnson & Johnson were fined billions for false advertising practices that directly contributed to the opiate crisis. Drug companies have made a fortune marketing prescription drugs to physicians and consumers with false promises. Focusing more on profit than healing, they have ignored the literature that shows many of these drugs are ineffective and highly addictive (Dragoo 2013, Jain 2018). It's called programming; we have been duped into believing medication is the key to resolve musculoskeletal pain. It's the by-product of years of marketing investment and the allure of the fix. Big Pharma has reaped huge financial rewards for direct marketing campaigns aimed at medical providers and consumers. Despite the risks of prescription drugs and recent research showing lack of benefit, prescriptions for expensive and highly addictive drugs continue to rise.

Each day, ninety Americans die prematurely from an overdose that involves an opioid (Rudd 2016). The burgeoning rates of addiction and death caused by drug abuse are directly related to the sharp rise of prescription opiates. Repeated studies have shown opiates and other types of controlled substances are highly addictive and lack effectiveness at improving function. Instead, prescription painkillers can worsen the painful response, making an individual more sensitive to pain (Dobrila-Dintinjana 2011, Garland 2019). This debunks the age-old claim of having a high tolerance for pain; if you take pain medications, then your tolerance for pain is markedly reduced due to the insatiable hunger the brain has for its opiate fix. It's a sad story shared by many clients. It starts with seeking a medical fix for pain, only to end up addicted to prescription pain medications.

Erika is a twenty-nine-year-old aspiring business manager with a history of chronic neck pain. She's always been a hard worker and avid runner, but lately the stress has been overwhelming. She has taken on a number of difficult accounts, which leaves her with little energy to exercise after work. About three months prior to coming to our clinic, she decided to get back into exercise. She admits overdoing it at the gym, and the next day she awoke with severe neck and upper back pain, leading her to visit her medical provider. She received a brief exam and follow-up imaging that showed some signs of degeneration. For her troubles, she was prescribed opiates and anti-inflammatory medication. She soon returned to work, and it seemed nearly impossible to make it through the daily stressors without pain medication. She lost any interest in exercise and activity. She simply went to work and recovered with meds. It wasn't long before she realized she was addicted to the pain medication. She tried multiple times to wean off the opiates, but the side effects were too debilitating. Finally, she went cold turkey and began physical therapy. She is now nearly pain-free, but insurance is denying coverage for more therapy. Interesting how the insurance never questioned or limited coverage of the medical fix, but conservative care is strictly limited. Unfortunately, this type of story is more common than expected. It is the typical example of how drugs have become the first line of response to musculoskeletal conditions. What's uncommon is the patient decided to become a health consumer, instead of a compliant patient, and took it upon herself to discontinue an addictive drug, making the choice to heal—not fix—the pain.

A brief summary of the frontline drugs for musculoskeletal pain should demonstrate why drugs should not be the first choice for musculoskeletal pain. The initial trials of many drugs are focused on a select spectrum or limited condition. Initially, the studies are too small and too short of a time frame to uncover all the drug-related risks. Long after the marketing tales have been spread, there is little attention to follow-up studies demonstrating significant side effects and risks that far outweigh the limited benefits. It's easy to assume that if a drug is legal and prescribed, then it must be safe. All drugs carry risks, and very few have worthwhile effects on tissue healing.

Classification	Drugs	Supporting evidence	Documented Risks
NSAIDs	Ibuprofen, Celebrex, Mobic, Meloxicam	Delays bone healing, detrimental effects on soft-tissue healing (7)	GI, CV, Renal dysfunction with long-term use
Anti-depressants	Cymbalta, Prozac, Lexapro, Paxil, Elavil	Failed to reduce pain with walking in knee OA (34). No better than placebo (23)	Common: Constipation, Dizziness, Erectile dysfunction, Insomnia, Uncommon: Suicide attempt, muscle spasms
Muscle Relaxants	Flexeril, Valium, Xanax	No significant effect on improving pain. No better than placebo (22)	Dizziness, Drowsiness, Depression, Fatigue, Decreased blood pressure
Opiates	Tramadol, Oxycotin, Hydrocodone, Percocet	Effective pain-relief for short-term use. Long-term use may increase pain sensitivity (32)	Addiction risk related to current opiate crisis proclaimed by the CDC
Anti-convulsants	Lyrica, Gabapentin	No significant effect. No better than placebo (30)	Angioedema, Dizziness, Weight gain, Suicide thoughts

Common drugs prescribed for musculoskeletal pain.

Surgery has become the preferred option to correct common musculoskeletal conditions. The prospect of surgery to address musculoskeletal dysfunction makes perfect sense from a structural standpoint. Surgeons are extremely talented in the diagnosis of structural problems. Their approach is to cut out (debride) or repair (suture or tack) the damaged tissue shown on imaging. However, if pain were entirely due to a structural problem, then the outcome of surgery would be absolute resolution of pain. Yet most procedures have a track record on par with placebo treatments. The painful reality is that function is often the primary cause of pain. The function of the entire musculoskeletal chain determines how structures are loaded within the movement system. Unfortunately, surgery is not capable of repairing function. Repair of the structure while leaving a dysfunction unchanged only leads back to tissue overload. It's like giving a chronic smoker a new lung. If he still smokes, then it's only a matter of time before the structure fails.

In full support of the overmedicalization of musculoskeletal conditions, Americans have been convinced it's possible to fix the structural problems found on imaging. Of course, there's little regard for the fact that functional tissue must be cut and removed to repair the structural problem. For instance, is it possible for a bone spur to cause pain? In a recent study of age-matched subjects with and without knee osteoarthritis (OA), the authors discovered similar findings on MRI for both groups. "Our findings highlight the great challenge in distinguishing pathological features of early knee OA from what could be considered part of 'normal aging'" (Kumm 2018). The reality is our method of justifying surgery by imaging is flawed. Degenerative changes in the tissue are often natural and only become painful when a functional imbalance causes tissue overload.

What about a disc herniation? Does it make sense to remove the big, fat disc bulge? Again, research shows that disc bulges are normal and very common in asymptomatic or nonpainful individuals. "On MRI examination of the lumbar spine, many people without back pain have disk bulges or protrusions..." Given the high prevalence of these findings, the discovery by MRI of bulges or protrusions in people with low back pain may be coincidental (Jensen 1994). It's just further justification for the two-sided story of musculo-skeletal pain. Blaming a structural problem, such as a disc herniation, for the cause of pain is like blaming the match for the fire. Someone had to light the match. Yes, structural problems like disc herniations are prone to be painful with improper loading, but it's the functional problems within the chain that cause the adverse tissue loading.

What about degraded cartilage like the meniscus? Once again, structural approaches like surgical debridement have been shown to be no better than a placebo. There is no better example of this notion than a recent study comparing outcomes on surgical repair versus placebo surgery (Sihvonen 2018). The subjects who received a placebo procedure (incisions for arthroscope but no meniscal repair) actually achieved better outcomes and more satisfaction than those receiving the typical meniscal repair surgery. This is the type of evidence that will remain ignored to allow hospitals to continue expansion of services. Just as prescription drugs have nearly doubled year after year, a similar trend can be found for surgical rates. All roads toward the fix lead to either drugs and (or) surgery. No country on the planet can hold a candle to the rates of drug prescription, imaging, or surgery in the United States. Sadly, none of these fix options treat the real cause or condition of musculoskeletal pain.

In most cases of musculoskeletal pain, the culprit is a gradual breakdown of tissue alliance rather than a single precipitating incident. Muscles and fascia form continuous pathways or loops of tension to support and move the skeletal chain. Loss of tissue alliance results when these loops fail to compensate for WIS, leading to imbalances in tissue loading. It's not the structure that's causing the pain; it's how tissue functions to load the structure. Attempting to correct a functional imbalance with a drug or surgical repair is shortsighted, with the risk far outweighing the potential reward. It simply masks or transfers the pain, creating a greater problem in the future. Any short-terms gains are likely achieved in part due to the high dose of pain relievers, surgical restrictions, and prolonged recovery after surgery.

How did the treatment of musculoskeletal pain become big business pushing the medical fix? A short walk back in history helps put the current pain crisis in perspective. It's tough to admit, but we've been duped before. As America was facing the greatest financial catastrophe of its history, the tobacco industry saw an opportunity to maximize profit. To achieve its goal of financial gain in the midst of the Great Depression, Big Tobacco ramped up marketing to squash rising concerns about the health effects of cigarette smoking. They had no qualms about hiding the truth and misleading the public with false ad campaigns. You would think we learned something from the smoking lie. Instead, a closer look at the most recent thirty-year trend of imaging, surgery, and drugs for musculoskeletal pain shows how we have been duped again.

Over the last few decades, we have witnessed a systematic collaboration among the biggest liars of the twenty-first century transforming health care into health business. In the areas of disease management, the health care system has justified the increased utilization of imaging, drugs, and surgery by saving lives from TIPS. However, in the case of musculoskeletal pain, overutilization of medical services has involved a coordinated pattern of lies to maximize profit and increase dependence. What lies are they spreading? "We care," "We help," and "We fix" are the three biggest lies of the twenty-first century. They are the favorite lies spread by the Big Three of health business: insurance, hospital, and drug corporations. It's a more complicated tale than the Big

Tobacco lie spun nearly a century ago, but the end-result is still driven by relentless corporate greed.

The lie of "We care" is spread by the insurance industry. It's standard practice for insurance companies to deny coverage for early conservative treatment of musculoskeletal conditions. Without any shame or regret, they are ignoring their solemn promise to the insured and discarding scientific literature showing the link between early treatment and prevention of disability. Why cover drugs or surgery as the primary fix for non-life-threatening conditions but deny conservative care that has been shown to reduce disability? It's easy if you look at it from a corporate standpoint. More chronic pain and higher risk of disability simply justifies the need for insurance coverage. No one wants to be left facing the high cost of health care without insurance. It's truly astounding how insurance companies are willing to push the medical fix agenda despite the risks to the insured. Rather than encouraging conservative treatment and wellness as the first response to musculoskeletal pain, the standard response is a path that leads to the fix. Insurers often require medical providers to order costly imaging to justify medical care. Unfortunately, it's common for the terrible images on x-ray or MRI to convince the patient that drugs and surgery are the only viable option for fixing their pain.

The reality is most people with musculoskeletal pain have little to no idea what led to their pain. Perhaps it was a string of events with sporadic bouts of pain and impaired function or a couple of minor trauma incidents that coalesced into a significant period of pain and inflammation. Often symptoms are poorly patterned, while functional limitations are more multifactorial than incidental. Using imaging to justify medical insurance coverage is lunacy, unless there was recent trauma or suspicion of pathology. Typically, the imaging study is determined by wherever the patient points to as being painful. However, just because the shoulder is painful does not mean the shoulder is the problem. The one consistent fact about musculoskeletal conditions is that the pain rarely occurs at the site of the problem.

The lie of "We help" is spread by the hospital industry. Our hospitals are some of the most advanced in the world. Whether it's responding to a world-wide crisis like COVID-19 or improving the health status of patients struggling with TIPS. Make no mistake, we are privileged to have the most advanced tools and talented medical teams in the world. Every hospital and the medical teams they employ do important and vital work. In all areas of disease and trauma management, the hospital is the place to get the right care. Still, even with all this technology and talent, it has become apparent that hospitals are not best suited to manage musculoskeletal pain.

Hospitals are the biggest employers of physicians and surgeons. They have immense operating costs due to huge facilities filled with expensive equipment and a vast number of specialists. Of course, the only way for these behemoth institutions to survive is revenue growth. This insatiable appetite for growth is magnified by the hospital monopoly. During the megamergers of the 1980s and 1990s, small- and large-scale medical facilities were gobbled up by corporations. Today, nearly two-thirds of the nation's hospitals are owned by a handful of corporate giants. Hospitals have truly become businesses that are too big to fail. Rather than trim and downsize to meet the needs of patients, they push for higher utilization of expensive imaging and risky surgeries. Rates of surgery have increased 126 percent for common procedures like total joint replacements and spinal fusion; that's 45 percent higher than any other country. The lack of any real competition and the need for constant revenue growth leaves hospitals unchecked to overmedicalize musculoskeletal conditions.

Lastly, the lie of "We fix" is spread by the pharmaceutical industry. Again, it's all about maximizing profits. This storyline borders on redundant, but there is no denying that drug corporations are the most profit driven of the Big Three. A recent lawsuit filed by forty-four states claims the nation's leading drug companies conspired to inflate the prices of generic drugs by as much as 1,000 percent. With their unlimited marketing budget, drug companies bombard American homes with ad campaigns designed to turn each American into a drug seeker. According to a 2017 Harris Poll, nearly half of Americans report to have taken prescription-based opioids, and about one in three Americans have personally experienced opioid dependency or abuse, whether it be themselves, a friend, or family member who has or is currently struggling. Nearly 70 percent of American adults are on at least one prescription medication, with anti-inflammatory medications being the most common. The reality is medications for pain and inflammation only treat the symptoms, not the problem. There is no drug designed to fix musculoskeletal dysfunction.

2
THE PAIN REVOLUTION

*You must be the change you
wish to see in the world.*
—GANDHI

Musculoskeletal conditions are the most common pain-related dysfunctions faced by Americans from adolescence to senior years. It wasn't long ago that Americans accepted pain and believed in healing. Remember the old adage, *no pain, no gain*, or one of my favorites, *rub some dirt on it*. Accepting pain and trusting healing have become less of a tradition with the high stakes of profit and litigation in today's health care system. Management of painful musculoskeletal dysfunctions has become a battleground. The campaign is waged by the Big Three using their favorite weapons: skyrocketing medical costs, legal pitfalls, and empty promises. This struggle has been waged for decades, while those suffering musculoskeletal pain wander from one camp to another in hopes of some relief.

For years, the Big Three have maintained the defining

edge as the experts directing the management of musculo-skeletal pain, but their stronghold is weakening. The stories of devastation and despair have become all too common. I recall the firefighter facing disability due to persistent back pain. He thought lumbar surgery was going to fix the herniated disc. Yet, after all the imaging and repeated trials of medication, spinal surgery failed to get him back to work. Just as shocking is the young real estate agent recovering from dependence on prescription painkillers. For years, she struggled with pain from whiplash, and now she struggles with drug addiction.

The Big Three have collaborated to remove the responsibility for recovery from the patient and place the burden on a system that is geared toward profit and expanding market share. It has become far too acceptable for the promise of hope and trust in healing to be supplanted by the profit of the health businesses. In every business, there is a commodity, something to wager and manipulate for the sole purpose of profit. In today's health business model, the commodity sold for profit is the independence and quality of life for patients. For far too long, people struggling with persistent musculoskeletal pain have been misguided by the Big Three to seek a fix. When patients become dependent on drugs or disabled due to mis/overtreatment of a musculoskeletal condition, that is not profit; it's a scam. Finally, the truth needs to be exposed. Any reliance upon the medical "fix" comes at a cost, and the results are often no better than placebo (Sihvonen 2018).

The unprecedented access to relevant research and healing options places us on a precipice for the pain revolution. Americans want and deserve better care for musculoskeletal pain. Science is readily available to anyone with a search option. It's uncovering a blatant fact: healing is still the best option for pain relief. Personal experience tells us that we are the only ones capable of restoring wellness. As we learn of natural and healthy choices to improve our wellness, there are endless opportunities to explore the most effective methods for healing.

My personal experience with musculoskeletal pain began during military deployment for Operation Desert Storm. It seems long ago, but pain tends to leave a mark on the psyche. During the haste of a military buildup, deployment of our small team of military police was riddled with mishaps. We had left our families and station, but we were stuck at an isolated transfer site, waiting for transport. I was tasked to get things moving and arrange transport for our team out of country. I was quick to jump at the chance; we were all anxious to leave the transit site and get into the action. Initially, I was surprised at how easy it was to arrange transport for our unit. Soon, I learned that my meager attempts would fail to squash this logistical nightmare. No sooner had I assured my team members that I had single-handedly resolved our transportation problems that some flaw in my plan would emerge. Initially, I arranged for us to piggyback on a flight with another unit. My proud moment was short-lived, as I was informed by higher command that there was no room for our gear. "Just guns and boots" was what their chief said. I went into full-blown scramble mode trying to arrange equipment transport to ensure gear and troops arrived in country on a similar time frame. At first try, I scored some space for our gear on a ship to Doha. Nearly perfect, except we were going to Camp Doha, Saudi Arabia, while the ship was going to Doha, Qatar. Easy mistake to make but a difficult foul-up for my team to accept. Undaunted, I reshuffled and arranged air transport for the gear. Of course, every change in transport required moving gear from shipping containers to airline pallets and then back again. I recruited a small team of volunteers from our team to help me out with the repeated transfer of gear. Unfortunately, my planning snafus with the transport of gear continued. My small team of volunteers became even smaller as suspicions grew that I was in over my head. Finally, just hours before our team was due to depart, I received the final solution for transport of our equipment. It would be sent by air, which meant everything had to be returned to pallets. I quickly roused my team, now dwindled down to just two other airmen, and began emptying the shipping containers of gear. I can still vividly remember being upset with my string of failures causing us to move the gear back and forth from container to pallets. Suddenly my back spasmed, and I fell to the ground after tossing a couple of heavy duffel bags. Never before had I experienced such excruciating pain. We still had pallets to pack, yet I simply could not move without triggering intense pain. Eventually, I stiffened up and recovered enough to assist my team. Still, I was frightened about the possible impact on my deployment and embarrassed by my limited movement, which had become obvious to my team. I feared I caused severe damage to my back and my life would never be the same. I was right about the latter, but it wasn't due to the back pain.

I'm sure everyone reading this book has their own memory of painful experiences. It's a harrowing experience to realize our body is not fully under our control. How simple movements cause severe pain, when normal activity hurts, where pain spreads to other regions—it all leaves us to question why. Musculoskeletal pain is quite unique since the problems occur gradually, making the onset of symptoms seem benign or strange despite the severity of pain. Pain can also develop with sudden onset due to awkward stress, leading to severe limits in function. Most of us have experienced pain in more than one form and various natures.

You would think with the widespread prevalence of muscu-loskeletal pain, every adult would have a basic knowledge of tissue-related pain and be aware of reasonable courses of action to achieve relief. Instead, it is this lack of healing knowledge that leads many people to seek a quick fix.

Understanding movement and tissue nutrition is the cru-cial step in determining what steps are necessary for turning painful problems into challenging opportunities. This is the struggle that has the potential to toughen or weaken the fabric of our lives. Many people struggle with the burden of musculoskeletal pain limiting every aspect of their daily lives. It's easy to wonder, *Why me?* but the real question is, *Why now?* The reality is that we are all one breath, one move, one effort, or one incident away from triggering pain. Searching for the why or cause of pain is a dangerous path towards the fix. Musculoskeletal pain deserves solutions and strategies, rather than disease-based labels. The cause is multifactorial, complex, and complicated. It's like trying to figure out where an emotional relationship went wrong. There's rarely one incident or event, instead it's a cascade of minor insults and imbalances which lead to failure of a system to perform at optimal levels. The movement system relies on every link to function at optimal levels of strength and balance. Pain is the primary method of communication between our awareness and movement. When movement and nutrition are not optimal to withstand loading, pain is the ping signaling an imbalance.

The pain revolution can only begin with individuals strik-ing out a new path toward recovery and pain relief. The path is readily available if we analyze the science in favor of healing and tear away the facade that suggests drugs and surgery are the only options. As our hope is restored in heal-ing, it becomes critical to accept personal responsibility for making changes that will improve wellness and activate the healing potential within the musculoskeletal system. Resist the ad campaigns and empty promises of the illusive fix and realize the amazing potential for healing in each well human.

With more than twenty-five years of clinical practice treating musculoskeletal pain, I have gained a unique insight into the challenges faced by clients struggling to find relief from musculoskeletal pain. Early in my profession, I adopted the medical model of pain that indicated pain as a sign of danger due to unhealthy or damaged tissue. With this limited perspective, my role as a physical therapist was to get patients moving. Motion is lotion. Start moving to get strong. This approach worked for some, but many patients still struggled with pain. Often, I assumed a lack of compliance or limited participation was the reason they failed to recover, despite my best efforts to offer evidence-based care. I believed "difficult patients" continued to experience pain because they were either incapable or not ready to heal. Such a narrow perspective failed to recognize the real healing potential of the human musculoskeletal system.

I have learned more from thousands of clients than any textbook. My failed attempt to help "difficult patients" recover from pain stemmed from disease-based assumptions and my inability to look beyond the painful site. If only I would have realized earlier what was known by Plato, "The cure of the part should not be attempted without treatment of the whole." Of course, I'm taking this quote out of context merely to appreciate the concept. Healing is a wholesome approach. What is healed is not restored to normal. It is simply made whole again, whereby the dysfunctional segment regains function (mobility, stability, and strength). Healing restores the ability of the musculoskeletal system to withstand physiological (normal) loads that are unavoidable in our daily lives.

Over time, I discovered the musculoskeletal system is

immensely resilient and capable of adapting despite significant structural deficits. I realized everyone wants and deserves to heal. I became convinced there is more to musculoskeletal pain than tissue damage and disease. Much of my musculoskeletal awakening was based upon my experience with clients and the opportunity to learn from a diverse group of healers. It's been a long journey as I tried different approaches to restore balance to a system dependent on movement and nutrition. I had to learn novel approaches to reassure clients that pain was not a threat but an opportunity. Most recently, I have discovered the importance of personal health and wellness to activate the healing potential. I am so thankful for my journey, and I hope to lighten your burden and struggle as either a pain sufferer or treatment provider.

The tools of a physical therapist are limited to hands-on techniques and reassurance. Out of this tool kit, it's easy to appreciate the complexities of human movement. In respect to the task-driven nervous system, all human movement occurs in harmony with a sole purpose: survival. Tissue restrictions are often adapted or imposed to allow survival as we struggle to withstand loading from daily activity. Impaired movements usually follow these dysfunctions as our ability to adapt and compensate is limited by tissue nutrition and general health. From treatment of clients with different degrees and stages of pain, it has become obvious that healing is not about getting it right. It's about respecting the whole person and the entire chain as movement and nutrition are restored to the tissue. It's equally important to resolve anxiety, frustration, and even depression through reassurance.

Simon is a retired air traffic controller with chronic LBP. He was becoming frustrated with pain keeping him from all the activities he planned to do in his retirement. His wife, Joan, had encouraged him to seek therapy since she had experienced success with treatment at our clinic. Joan was involved in a devastating motor vehicle accident that caused multiple injuries and significant pain. She was vested 100 percent in her healing and readily implemented suggestions to improve her wellness. She took steps to reduce screen time at night, which allowed her to get at least six to seven hours of restful sleep each night. She joined friends for daily walking and participated in a group exercise program. Her spirits were high, and she was excited with her recent weight loss from eating healthy. On the other hand, Simon was a bit reluctant to make changes to improve his wellness.

He was unable to see how minor changes could impact his severe back condition, referring to the MRI findings of disc degeneration. He continued to remain sleep-deprived, inactive, overweight, and depressed throughout therapy. His pain resulted in a drastic avoidance of activity, while he continued to maintain poor habits in critical areas of wellness. It was a real eye-opener to watch one client excel with healing and pain relief, while the other continued to decline in health and worsening symptoms. Joan triggered her healing potential, allowing her a speedy recovery from diffuse joint pain, while Simon hit the tissue barrier where recurrent patterns of pain and limited function weighed him down, thus limiting options for restoring wellness. Unfortunately, he continued to choose the fix-it approach and recently returned to therapy after another surgical procedure. This time it was a tendon tear in the lower leg. Finally, he is coming around to understand that wellness is the missing link to activate healing potential. It will require significant time and changes to improve his wellness, but it's never too late to activate healing potential.

Pain is a driving force to realize our responsibility for improving wellness. If you can harness the power of pain rather than avoid it altogether, there's no limit to what you can achieve. Wellness is entirely within our reach. Putting a priority on how we fuel our body with sleep, activity, fitness, and eating (SAFE) is critical to maintaining health of the musculoskeletal system with wellness safety. Oftentimes, it is the primary factor for maintaining tissue health. The musculoskeletal system is like a battery that must be recharged on daily basis. Wellness is the docking station for our tissue, giving it the rest and power to thrive. It is the key to unlocking the healing potential with movement and tissue nutrition. Putting these principles into action makes you an active participant in the pain revolution.

3

WELLNESS SAFE

*When you're finished
changing, you're finished.*
—BENJAMIN FRANKLIN

There is valid scientific evidence that supports certain elements of lifestyle as essential pillars of wellness. Wellness is the quality or state of being in good health especially as an actively sought goal. It involves lifestyle choices and habits which fosters quality of life by taking action and making changes to improve health. Wellness is the sum of our choices and behaviors as we struggle to make a difference in our life and the lives of others.

A good dose of sleep and activity keeps the mind fit and the body healthy if it's fueled by good nutrition. In fact, these same behaviors that have been proven to reduce the risk for disease can also improve musculoskeletal health and support healing. For instance, impaired sleep patterns have been shown to increase the risk for nearly all musculoskeletal dysfunctions and many diseases (Smith 2004). Improving sleep hygiene restores tissue nutrition to more optimal levels. Consider the role of activity, sedentary lifestyles are associated with increased mortality rates (Buchman 2010). Variable activity and aerobic exercise replenish tissue strength and endurance. Probably one of the most challenging areas to address in wellness is fitness of mind and spirit. It is quite common for chronic pain to be accompanied by depression (Abdallah 2017). The current trend is to explain and recondition the pain perception, but there may be other options that simply restore hope and joy. Nutrition is the simplest way to access healing potential. Rather than writing a referral for imaging or medication, most clients would be better served to complete an inventory of their wellness safe to identify areas for improvement.

The pillars of wellness are based on creating homeostasis, which allows the body to self-repair and adapt to change. Musculoskeletal pain is more often caused by tissue overload than physical injury; instead of inflammation, it is more related to imbalances. In the case of musculoskeletal conditions, pain is not a sign of injury; it's a signal of opportunity—opportunities to correct movement and restore balance that will trigger the nervous system to release healing potential and restore balance to dysfunctional tissues. Thanks to the science revolution, there are hidden gems and precise steps to guide our efforts toward finding the most likely areas involved in delayed healing and persistent musculoskeletal pain.

Wellness is something we all desire but rarely achieve. It is life in balance with nature and community. In short, it is health maintenance. Just like pain fuels change, wellness fuels healing. We live in a tough and ruthless world based upon consumption and convenience. The success of our work is represented by what we own, while our means for survival are geared toward convenience. We no longer have to rip our food out of the ground or drag our meal to the table. Thankfully, we have all the conveniences of the twenty-first century, but it comes at a cost.

Americans are more inactive than any other time in history. According to the American Heart Association, sedentary jobs have increased by 83 percent since 1950. This explains the most recent data from the Centers of Disease Control and Prevention showing more than one-third of adults in the US are obese. Our struggle to survive has been restricted to sitting and interacting with screens rather than people. Even worse, our main form of entertainment and interaction has become digital, thus making us more isolated and stifling our need to struggle. I'm no psychologist, but it's pretty obvious we have become far removed from our struggle for survival due to sedentary work and lack of community. For many experiencing pain, the tendency for less activity and isolation from others is a real problem. Challenge your body and mind with survival and positive relationships.

The pillars of wellness are deeply interdependent and relative to healing. It's tough maintaining physical well-being without an active lifestyle. It's even tougher to gain mental wellness while lacking any sense of connection or community. Wellness doesn't require us to be an elite athlete or social butterfly, but it does require attention to responsible actions to keep our health safe from disease and dysfunction. These healthy lifestyle choices are summed up in the Wellness SAFE.

SAFE pillars of Wellness include the following:
Sleep Well: Get at least six to seven hours of sleep each night.
Active Body: Variable activity on daily basis to live well.
Fit Soul: Seek peace of mind and spirit to feel well.
Eat Well: Choose a moderate and balanced diet while avoiding unhealthy habits.

Don't make the mistake of avoiding wellness flaws just because the changes seem out of reach or too daunting. Perfection is not our goal; your nervous system will make use of the slightest improvements to improve musculo-skeletal health and aid healing. There's no need to have a perfect Wellness SAFE, since gains made in any of the pillars can set the environment for healing. I've come across all kinds of healers. Some are poor in spirit, yet they heal if they have some consistency in good sleep patterns and regular activity. Others may not have the best diet, but they have a great attitude and exercise routinely. You can be well without being perfect, but there must be some overall level of wellness to achieve healing. If we look at persistent musculoskeletal pain as an opportunity, the opportunity starts with improving one or more pillars to improve your Wellness SAFE.

SAFE: Sleep Is the Body's Mechanic

At the end of a difficult day, sleep is a welcome release. A good night's sleep is credited with restoring healthy brain function and physical well-being. Basically, the way you feel when you're awake depends on how well you sleep. Disturbed sleep is often due to various stressors, with the most common reported being persistent pain, depression, and (or) anxiety. More than 35 percent of adults are not getting enough sleep on a regular basis (CDC). The American Academy of Sleep Medicine and the Sleep Research Society recommend that adults sleep at least seven hours each night to promote optimal health and well-being. Sleeping less than seven hours is associated with an increased risk of developing chronic conditions, such as obesity, diabetes, high blood pressure, heart disease, stroke, and frequent mental distress (Kim 2013).

Sleep activates the human body mechanic. Every system of the human body depends on sleep to make vital repairs. Getting the right amount of sleep activates healing potential and enhances tissue nutrition. You could argue that more pain means less sleep, but the evidence points in the opposite direction. Experimental studies of healthy subjects suggest that poor sleep further exacerbates pain (Smith 2004). Sleep helps your brain form new pathways to learn skills and remember information, thus causing less stress. It even helps you make better decisions and improves your problem-solving skills. Sleep sets the stage for improved mood and a positive outlook, so it's time to sleep well.

Sleep Well *(ABC)*: Implement principles of good sleep hygiene to ensure tissue recovery.
- *Alignment* is a priority when choosing the best support. Whether it's the fluff of your pillow or firmness of the mattress, it should encourage symmetry and unloading.
- *Breathing* is an important consideration for sleeping position. Many adults struggle with impaired breathing during sleep due to obstructive sleep apnea. This affliction of oral motor (tongue and jaw muscles) weakness is more pronounced with sleeping flat on the back.
- *Comfort* is critical for any support. It's tough to claim one surface is better than another (gel versus air versus springs), but the true measure is the surface that provides the best perceived comfort.

Sleep is a behavior, not an identity. Most of us have experienced some sleepless nights, but it is important not to accept disturbed sleep as the norm. Whether it's recovery from surgery or healing from a chronic injury, sleep is a necessary element of the healing process (Vanini 2016). Once we have emerged alive and awake from the tissue trauma, the long journey ahead is far less difficult if we develop good sleep behaviors. Sleep is even more crucial for the health of the musculoskeletal system. The human body needs rest to recover from tissue overload and replenish tissue nutrition. Sleep.org and Sleepopolis.com offer some excellent resources on improving sleep habits.

SAFE: **Activity Is a Necessity**
Activity is the fuel for the human experience. Variable levels of activity throughout each day help the major body systems maintain health. It is important to choose activities that unravel the stiffness in vessels (blood and nerve) and restore strength and endurance. Unfortunately, for many of us, static postures have become the norm. Just consider briefly how much of your day is dedicated to downtime, particularly sitting. You sit for the long commute, then sit at work, followed by another period of commuting home, only to sit and relax because a sedentary life is simply exhausting. Static postures pose enormous health risks and trigger fatigue and exhaustion (Daneshmandi 2017). According to the Mayo Clinic, prolonged periods of sitting carry the same mortality risks as obesity and smoking. If your day involves prolonged periods of static posture, then you face an uphill battle to regain wellness. You only get the energy that you bank, so it's important to make a deposit each day. Pay back the energy used to accomplish your life's work.

Having a physical and labor-intensive job does not void the need for variable activity. Oftentimes, I'll get a client who claims they get enough exercise at work. If their point was valid, then competitive athletes are spending way too much time exercising. A more physical job challenges your musculoskeletal system to function at optimal levels of performance. The risk for injury is high if you fail to replenish strength and endurance on a daily basis. It's convenient in the form of physical exertion, but many segments of the musculoskeletal chain are exposed to tissue overload from misuse, overuse, or disuse (MOD). Consider how much of your physical exertion is dedicated to one plane of movement. For instance, go to any gym, and you'll find most people exercising on equipment that only challenges muscles in the sagittal plane (front to back). You have to be creative to spend time working in the other two planes (frontal and transverse) to truly challenge the musculoskeletal chain in all three dimensions. The tendency to operate in one or two dimensions of motion leaves muscles and joints in the less utilized plane of motion subject to functional imbalances (WIS). The presence of weakness or instability particularly in the frontal and transverse planes has been shown to increase risks for athletic injuries (Mosher 2004). The traditional military notion, *train as you fight, fight as you train*, is a relevant motto for today's industrial athlete.

With today's growing trend for convenience and desensitization, it's important to keep our musculoskeletal chains healthy and our minds alert. If your daily activity is limited due to sedentary work setting, then it's time to invest some sweat equity to restore tissue health. If you are active at work and play, then it's important to achieve optimal function in all three dimensions of movement by novel exercises to weed out WIS and restore optimal tension in the myofascial loops. Regardless of which group you fall into, it's important to consider the side benefit of variable physical activity. Choose either a fifteen-minute brisk walk or six-minute leisure run to improve physical fitness and ward off the dangerous health risks of inactivity (Lee 2014).

Act Well *(DEF)*: Implement principles of an active lifestyle to improve tissue resilience.

- *Daily* activity is necessary to counter the effects of prolonged postures and repetitive loads. If static postures are part of your work, then be active for at least one hour each day. If you primarily work in one or two dimensions, then add variable movements to challenge stability.
- *Endurance* is a necessary element for variable levels of activity. Sweat it out; it's the best way to increase tissue nutrition by increasing demand for vascularization of the deep tissues.
- *Fitness* achieves a balance of strength and endurance. Replenish the strength and endurance necessary to keep the musculoskeletal system healthy. Try out a group exercise class or do a progressive strength routine at home.

Physical activity restores our drive for knowledge, discovery, and arousal, which is easily dampened by the abundance of useless information, mundane tasks, and sterile interactions. When was your last great adventure? What have you recently discovered? Being active in body and mind requires new movement patterns and skill building. Try a fitness class, train for a 5k run, learn a new sport or exercise routine. As time passes, you will regain your sharp edge, and movements will be less painful. Don't let your drive for an active life be stifled by pain. Our movement system desperately needs stimulation, which comes in the form of three-dimensional motion and skilled activity.

SAFE: **Fitness of the Soul**
Fitness of mind and spirit is where so many of us struggle. We don't have to walk around all day with a smile plastered on our face, although smiling and laughing are great ways to achieve mental fitness (Bennett 2003). If you are struggling with emotional pain, then it's important to begin the slow process of rebuilding relationships and restoring trust. Musculoskeletal pain is directly influenced by our mental and emotional fitness. Struggles with anger and anxiety will only heighten pain awareness. General well-being and health are compromised by depression and despair. If you seek less physical pain, then it's time to get some peace of mind and joy of spirit.

The mind is a powerful pain reliever. It's possible that pain can be controlled merely with our thoughts. A recent study on the use of mindfulness-oriented recovery enhancement (MORE) demonstrated the power of being present and mindful (Garland 2019). The study recruited 135 chronic pain sufferers with prolonged opiate usage. After an eight-week MORE treatment program, the participants showed the ability to reduce reliance on opiates. Mindfulness is defined as paying attention to the present moment, without judgment. It involves taking a pause in our busy lives to reflect and enhance our awareness of our present feelings, thoughts, and reality, all while accepting the fact that judgment is pointless.

The best route to changing pain perception and fear-avoidance behaviors is far simpler than we imagine. Rather than trying to convince clients that pain is not so bad, or struggle with trying to find the origin of pain, it's more worthwhile to be mindful and enjoy movement. Playing around with movement is a simple way to explore movement with emphasis on the task rather than the pain. Have fun with exercise and incorporate timing and accuracy of movement to interrupt the perception that movement is harmful.

Feel Well *(GHI)*: It takes practice and determination to create an internal healing environment.
- *Grace* is a shared gift within our community. We judge no one and expect not to be judged.
- *Hope* is our basis for belief and trust in others. Hope is the secret ingredient to happiness.
- *Inspire* others by your life and struggle. Build up your neighbors and community.

More importantly, it's necessary to develop your own peace and hope. Make peace with yourself and others. Spread hope with trust and faith in the common goodness that exists in all of us. Stop shooting down your own dreams. I can't tell you how many times I nearly failed to complete this book. I tried to convince myself it was too informative, not entertaining enough, and frankly just not worth the effort. But I had a dream, and it took heart and the support of others to put it into action. There is no harm done in making a dream come true. If you can't imagine putting your own dreams into action, then help someone else see their dreams become a reality. You don't have to be gifted; just invest some time and support to make your community better. It will do your soul well to care for yourself as you would for others.

SAFE: Eating for Success

A healthy and nutritious diet is essential to a person's well-being. These days, everyone seems to be an expert on nutrition; in some ways, that may be a bonus. We understand the importance of eating a balanced diet and avoiding too much processed food. But an overbearing emphasis on nutrition could also be a curse. It seems there are so many versions of the proper diet that it's nearly impossible to determine the right path. We eat for more reasons than just nutrition. Eating is part of our communion with family and friends. It's how we explore new tastes and cultures. It may be even how we show our love. I still remember visiting my wife's parents for the first time. I was served a big bowl of seafood gumbo, which seemed to have more sand than seafood. Thankfully, my wife found a way to get me excused from the table but only after finishing my third bowl. Some reasons for why we eat simply don't make sense to anyone other than those we love.

Nutrition is one area where there are too many experts and not enough consensus. Rather than stressing about eating the right foods, consider how and why you eat. Eat only what you need to fuel your day. Develop healthy relationships with friends and family that don't always include eating. There is no need to fret over expensive organics and useless supplements. Just keep your diet practical and natural and practice moderation. For the latest science on nutrition, check out the Nutrition Facts website (nutritionfacts.org).

Eat Well *(JKL)*: Nutrition is our life source and fuel for tissue buildup (strength and stability).
- *Junk* food is out.
- *Keep* it balanced and unprocessed.
- *Limit* intake of fat and sugar.

Often, I will expand the Wellness SAFE to be more about SAFETY. Yes, it's important to have a routine sleep pattern, active lifestyle, and fit mind all while eating healthy. It's also important to keep in mind that change takes time, so be patient. More importantly, health and lifestyle changes require your commitment and willingness to eliminate bad habits. If you have more than just a couple of areas of wellness that require improvement, then consider the broader approach of Wellness SAFETY.

SAFETY: Change takes time; be patient and pace yourself. The longer it's been, the more time needed to reclaim wellness. If it's been a while since you've been active, then respect the slow transition from sedentary to active lifestyle. It's likely that new bouts of activity will cause muscle fatigue and soreness but hurt does not always equal harm. Often if we use variable activity to prevent muscle fatigue and soreness, it allows our body to recover more quickly. So don't quit just because you hurt; simply try a different activity and keep driving on. Trying to achieve some peace for fitness of mind and spirit requires small changes in attitude and perspective. Remember the best way to help yourself is to help someone else. Most of us will struggle with healthy nutrition throughout our lives. Don't make sudden changes that are unsustainable. Eat healthy snacks, drink lots of water, and begin changing out the cupboards with healthier choices. Finally, none of these changes matter if you fail to address the number one determinant of health and wellness: sleep. You must make changes to achieve optimal sleep since this is the only time your body can access the repair mechanisms of healing.

SAFETY: You hold the key.
It's possible you are your worst enemy when it comes to wellness. Some habits have a negligible effect on wellness, while others are truly harmful. The most dangerous impact on your health comes from addictive substances. Drugs such as, alcohol, tobacco, and opiates have no place in the healing process. If you can't quit, then you are essentially accepting a limited chance at recovery. There is no alternative to cessation; these habits directly impact healing by reducing the tissue nutrition necessary for healing. Now is the time to establish a new habit to rid yourself of these harmful behaviors.

Little do we realize how much of our activity and behavior is controlled by habits. Some habits build a better Wellness SAFE, while others can destroy it. According to the book *The Power of Habit* by Charles Duhigg, our habits follow a loop. The "Habit Loop" starts with a cue and ends with a satisfaction or reward. The key to eliminating bad or destructive habits is to replace them with a good habit. Start a habit loop of eating a piece of dark chocolate after a meal, instead of smoking. Rather than the fake reward of nicotine in your system, you'll get the real benefit of sweet antioxidants and minerals lowering the risk for heart disease.

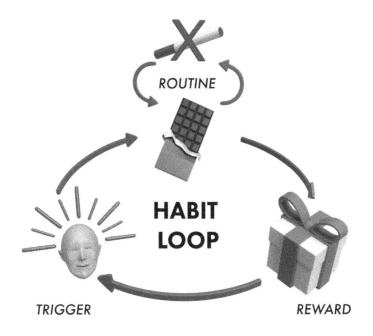

ROUTINE

HABIT LOOP

TRIGGER   *REWARD*

Every well human moves to heal. Wellness is not genetic, nor is it guaranteed. It's a life source that becomes available to each person willing to restore some balance to their lives and have a positive impact on their community. Without wellness, your healing potential is drastically reduced. If you want to avoid the fix and resolve musculoskeletal pain naturally, then wellness is your first step toward healing. Fortunately, all elements of the Wellness SAFE are interdependent. It's no use trying to focus on just one aspect; nutrition fuels activity, while activity warrants sleep and fitness of soul gives us peace to accept that we are not perfect, and change takes time.

If you are suffering from musculoskeletal pain, it's time to take an inventory of your Wellness SAFE and initiate changes for natural healing and pain relief. If you are a practitioner, then you have a responsibility to learn the pillars of wellness and guide patients toward improved health to establish a foundation for healing. Simon decided to take inventory of his Wellness SAFE. Needless to say, he has areas that may require drastic changes to improve health and establish a foundation for healing. Fortunately, he has plenty of time and motivation to make the necessary changes and lifestyle adjustments. Plus, he has the support of family and friends. We know his sleep pattern is very disruptive since he struggles with sleep apnea and likes to watch old movies before bed. Also, he dedicates little to no time for exercise, and his diet is lacking healthy snacks. Still, he maintains healthy relationships with family and friends.

Simon's Wellness Inventory:
Sleep: Less than six hours of consecutive sleep.
Activity: No routine aerobic exercise.
Fitness: No significant stressors affecting relationships.
Eating: Diet lacks fruits and vegetables and includes junk food snacking.

During the next visit, Simon agreed that serious changes were necessary to improve his Wellness SAFE. He outlined some habit loops to address each pillar of wellness and set a timeline for reassessment. Within a couple months, he was already experiencing less pain, and his surgery recovery was progressing well. He was so pleased with the treatment he received that he claimed, "You guys work magic." Personally, I think Simon made more progress due to his improved Wellness SAFE, but we'll settle with sharing the credit.

Visit www.newak.com for tutorials on Wellness SAFE and take your own inventory.

4 CHAINS AND LOOPS

Healing flows through movement.
—KEITH

The musculoskeletal system is often referred to as a chain. It does involve a series of joints and muscles that are connected from one segment to the next, similar to a chain with multiple links. Yet something is lacking in this description. The majority of the connections within the movement system involve soft rather than hard bony attachments. Rather than rigid links in a chain, the connections form mobile pathways of tension. In fact, nearly 80 percent of the tensile connections involve an alliance with muscles, fascia, ligaments, and capsules. That means bony connections make up less than one quarter of the attachments within the musculoskeletal system. It's true, a chain does not move itself; there must be some force or tension to turn the gears.

Myofascial tension is generated along concise direction-specific paths to create a region of stability while still allowing freedom of movement. This description is far more complex than generalizations made in anatomy textbooks, where muscles are simply depicted as bony attachments. Muscles and fascia work together to create a balance of myofascial tension that powers the musculoskeletal chain. It's not just about force or torque; it's about creating a stable and mobile movement system. Muscles are connected along a well-defined route where bands of fascia wrap and envelop nearly every muscular component from fibers to bundles, creating a pathway of tension. Since pathway of tension is too lengthy and chains are more relevant to the musculoskeletal system as a whole, my preference is to use the term myofascial loops. In my clinical experience, it simply makes sense to explain dysfunction and healing in relation to myofascial loops. A chain can't shorten, bend, or twist. Nor does a problem at one link of the chain imply that a restriction can be expected at the opposing side. Myofascial loops are synonymous with myofascial chains; I just prefer the former as a more definitive description of myofascial tension.

Myofascial loops are activated in a manner that has been repeatedly practiced and reinforced by the nervous system to allow the musculoskeletal chain to efficiently move and respond to loading. Myofascial loops involve the concise activation of muscles along a specific fascial plane, synchronized by the nervous system to create functional stability and movement throughout the musculoskeletal chain to withstand loading. These loops provide overlapping support from proximal to distal along the entire chain. Myofascial loops represent a system of force generation and shock absorption that is neurologically synced to respond to loading in an efficient and task-oriented manner.

Myofascial loops are the functional components of the musculoskeletal chain. These continuous loops of tension work in series from head to heel and side to side. Each loop is arranged to withstand loading and generate movement in three-dimensional positions and tasks. This requires an integrated and interconnected system that has opposing sides dependent upon strength, stability, and freedom of movement. Myofascial loops are the primary movers and torque producers of the human movement system. Optimal function of the myofascial loops allows us to move in a precise and coordinated fashion without risk of tissue overload. Nothing happens in isolation within this tension-based movement system. Thus, an imbalance anywhere within the chain or along the paths in the loops can trigger altered movement patterns and risk tissue overload.

Myofascial loops travel either front to back (sagittal loop), side to side (frontal loop), or across (oblique loop) the musculoskeletal chain. These 3D paths of tension are hardwired by the nervous system to easily adapt to movement restrictions to maintain stability and mobility with the least amount of effort. The highly neural-tuned movement strategies are developed over time, but compensatory changes occur due to segmental restrictions caused by structural deficits or functional impairments. Structural limits such as narrowed joint space or capsular stiffness will be accompanied by altered tension in the supporting myofascial loops. Typically, the primary response is a combination of dimensional weakness and stiffness throughout the loop. Functional impairments of weakness, instability, or stiffness (WIS) may cause an entire myofascial loop to become tangled. Even so, it's important to look beyond the pain or limit. For instance, hip flexor weakness won't be resolved by simply strengthening the hip. Instead, freedom of movement must be restored throughout the entire sagittal loop to regain a balance of strength and stability in the chain.

Optimal function of the myofascial loops center and align

skeletal joints with compression while balancing tension to create movement in a nearly friction-free fashion. The myofascial loops are driven by the nervous system to create just the right amount of compression to facilitate joint stability while harnessing tension to generate movement and force. All movement is achieved through a balance of joint stability and tissue mobility. More importantly, myofascial loops balance tension to withstand tissue loading within the musculoskeletal chain. Achieving this balance is a constant struggle in the presence of functional limitations (WIS) that may exist throughout the musculoskeletal chain.

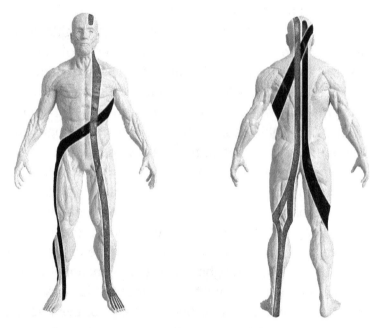

Illustration of Myofascial Loops: Light path: Sagittal loop / Dark path: Oblique loop

Movement is not an event; it's the integration of stability and mobility in response to loading while maintaining the ability to generate force. As one region is moving, another region must prepare for the movement with a dimension of stability. Why is this important? Essentially, it proves that dysfunction (WIS) is rarely located at the painful site. Myofascial loops generate tension across entire regions of the chain to produce movement and respond to loading. Rather than supporting a single segment, these loops operate in a broad fashion to prepare the chain for loading while still maintaining mobility and balance. The myofascial loops function as either mobile stabilizers or stabile mobilizers of the chain, which makes it quite rare for tissue overload to occur at the site of dysfunction.

It's continuous and interdependent. Movement of the human body is a balanced interaction of tension along all the myofascial loops. If one myofascial loop has a few dysfunctional segments (WIS), then it will affect the force production and transmission along the entire musculoskeletal chain, which increases the risk for tissue overload. Like trying to close a stuck drawer, if you continue to push it closed, something could be overloaded and become irritated. Instead, if you adjust and adapt to compensate for the restriction, then the drawer slides shut. This is similar to how our body compensates for WIS in the myofascial loops. Just like our mind and spirit are not always functioning at optimal levels, the same is true for the movement system. There is always some form of compensatory movement or altered posture due to segmental dysfunction. If these become persistent, then the tissue overload can develop and lead to a cycle of pain and inflammation at a site that is already degenerated or impaired.

The presence of inflammation is not the only determinant of pain. If tissue nutrition is sufficient, it's possible to avoid pooling of waste cells, which often occurs around overloaded tissue. This is why movement is of vital importance to flush out the inflammation and restore nutrition to the tissue. In absence of inflammation, pain may still occur due to the imbalance of tissue loading. Noninflammatory pain occurs due to the anisotropic nature of soft tissue. I'm not a fan of fancy words, but anisotropic really sums up how collagen responds to load in a manner specific to the direction of force or load. For instance, muscle and fascia readily absorb tensile force, while compression leads to overload and strain. The opposite is true for cartilage; it is designed to withstand compression, while shear and tension causes overload and failure. Tissue overload is dependent upon the anisotropic properties of the tissue being compromised and the frequency of impaired loading. The combination of awkward movements with improper loading may lead to misuse causing shear stress to cartilage and bone. Repetitive loads can cause overuse of tensile structures while lack of loading can lead to disuse. Misuse, overuse, disuse (MOD) are the main forms of tissue overload that often lead to musculoskeletal pain regardless of whether inflammation is present or not.

The musculoskeletal chain and myofascial loops form the framework of flow and movement. Flow of nutrition and conduction occurs through the myofascial layers to maintain tissue gliding and hydration. Blood and nerve vessels travel together as neurovascular bundles coursing through the layers of muscles and pierce the fascia to reach terminal points in the joints and soft tissues. Static postures and sedentary lifestyle put this nutrition flow at risk. Reduced activity or lack of movement variability makes it difficult for the musculoskeletal chain to respond to loading and impairs healing potential. Neurovascular flow directly impacts tissue alliance that is vital for optimal tissue nutrition and activation of myofascial tension. For instance, impaired flow is a more likely culprit for nerve problems like sciatica. The disease-based approach blames nerve irritations on structural lesions such as bone spurs or herniated discs causing a pinched nerve. Yet the nerves travel their entire length along myofascial passages, which poses a greater risk for tissue overload (MOD), leading to impaired flow. The beauty of this explanation for nerve problems is it helps us appreciate that no fix is required. We simply have to restore flow and movement. Improved movement and flow along the myofascial loops allow vital nutrition and nerve conduction to be restored, which will activate healing potential along the nerve pathways.

It's difficult to appreciate the whole when a part hurts. All too often, the tendency is to focus on the area that is painful. It's not immediately apparent to someone with knee pain to consider whether they have been practicing adequate wellness. Nor would they imagine that weak hip muscles or ankle instability could either impair healing or be the primary cause of knee pain. Yet this is exactly how we should approach musculoskeletal pain. Treating just the painful part is like punishing bad behavior without considering the cause. The musculoskeletal chain serves as the fundamental basis for the human movement system. Since movement of one region is dependent upon strength and stability of other regions, the whole is more important than the part.

If we could validate and prove the musculoskeletal system consists of an interconnected chain that is primarily anchored by connective tissue rather than bone, it would put the medical model into a tailspin. Actually, this proof already exists in the form of the most stringent and valid forms of research. A systematic review of sixty-two peer-reviewed research articles made the following determination: Fascia connects the skeletal muscles, forming a body-wide web of myofascial tension (Wilke 2016). The authors describe the existence of five myofascial chains in the human body. It was concluded that most skeletal muscles of the human body are directly linked by connective tissue. Obviously, this article did not garner much attention by the medical system since pain is still considered a local problem rather than a chain-related problem. The relevance of this finding has largely been ignored since it explains two important factors regarding musculoskeletal pain. First, the existence of a body-wide web of myofascial tension helps to explain why the problem is rarely located at the painful area. Second, direct continuity between muscles and fascia provides the justification to examine and treat beyond a single anatomic structure (Stecco 2009).

Loading creates tissue changes over time. After the age of twenty-five, joints and soft tissue are gradually breaking down rather than building up. The movement system does not age gracefully. Degenerative changes are natural and expected, but the onset of pain is based on more than just structure. Degeneration may set the stage for musculoskeletal pain, but it is not the main act. Once structural deficits are coupled with functional imbalances in strength, stability, or mobility, the process of tissue overload often leads to pain and inflammation. Function is immensely critical within the movement system, perhaps even more so than structure. In fact, many structural deficits actually develop due to a functional imbalance. Bone spurs at the heel or loss of joint space (arthrosis) at the knee actually develop as an age-related response to tissue overload caused by weakness of the locomotor muscles (i.e., gluteal and gastrocnemius). Other examples of function affecting structure include functional instability leading to disc lesions, while functional stiffness precedes spinal stenosis. Essentially, the presence of functional imbalances (WIS) predispose nearby structures to degeneration and injury. Recent evidence has shown weakness in the hip muscles can lead to ligament tears in the knee (Khayambashi 2015, Verrelst 2018). Maintaining optimal mobility, stability, and strength of the chain and loops allows function to compensate for structural deficits. Optimal tissue function can even be a deterrent to the onset or progression of degeneration. Maintaining a moderate level of wellness and optimal fitness defends against injury and activates healing potential throughout the entire musculoskeletal chain.

If we consider the interdependence of structure and function in the musculoskeletal chain, it's easier to appreciate pain as an opportunity, rather than a sign of danger. In reality, musculoskeletal pain is simply a message or maybe a real thorn in our side telling us it's high time to create change— changes in habits to become healthy and well, changes in behavior to improve fitness, and changes in movement to facilitate more balance and mobility. Some of these changes require attention to behaviors that can improve wellness, while changes in movement are necessary to activate healing potential to restore functional balance and correct movement patterns.

There is no normal when it comes to tissue overload. Dysfunction (WIS) in one or more segments, whether it's a joint or tissue restriction, leads to altered movement patterns and impaired load tolerance throughout the entire movement system. Whether it's loading from sustained postures, repeated activity, or awkward movements, the outcome is the same. The musculoskeletal parts are connected from heel to head to allow movement and withstand physiological loading. Any deviation from the preferred loading pattern can lead to tissue overload in the form of misuse, overuse, or disuse (MOD). Tissue overload sets the stage for pain and inflammation. Once the pain cycle begins, changes are necessary to restore balance of tension to reduce or eliminate tissue overload.

Every segment in the chain and path of the loops is

affected to some degree once the cycle of pain and inflammation is triggered. This is the confounding nature of a chain and loop dysfunction; there is no pain without compensatory movement and altered myofascial tension. Hence the problem exists above and below the painful site, from front to back, or side to side. Low back pain is traditionally managed with treatment focused at the painful region of the back. If we use a chain and loop approach, it's more important to identify dysfunctions present at the thoracic region and hips, not just at the back, but along the front and sides of the trunk. Working around the pain, rather than at the pain, creates an opportunity for the nervous system to access the change in tissue movement and blood flow. Treat the chain and loops to heal pain. This comprehensive approach restores balance to the entire movement system rather than simply creating a distraction at the site of pain. There are lots of distractions out there, from simple foam rolling to complex methods of taping. Distractions may resolve some local pain, but there's no real effect on the dysfunctions (WIS) contributing to tissue overload (MOD).

Tissue overload is often accompanied by some form of impaired movement or inadequate myofascial tension leading to compensation throughout the chain and loops. The only option for dampening a functional imbalance is to address the segmental dysfunction (WIS) wherever it exists. This comprehensive approach has allowed me to discover that dysfunction and pain are rarely located at the same area. Resolving dysfunction in the musculoskeletal chain and myofascial loops is the key to unlocking healing potential. Pain-altered movement strategies require a progressive challenge of positional awareness and skilled movement to retrain normal movement patterns. Functional limits (WIS) in the myofascial loops require progressive tissue loading with variability in support, symmetry, and stability to restore optimal myofascial tension in all three dimensions. Unpacking the nature of our healing potential makes seeking a quick fix pointless.

Healing restores the load ability of tissue by improving balance of tissue mobility, strength, and stability throughout the entire musculoskeletal chain. This is the type of healing that should be the first choice for treatment of musculoskeletal pain. It's time we face the reality; drugs and surgery will never fix the cause(s) of musculoskeletal pain. There is no replacement for healing, drugs only mask the pain, and procedures simply shift the tissue overload elsewhere, creating the potential for another disorder in the future. I recall a bit of advice I received from a client. She explained, "Life is school, and failures are simply part of the lesson plan." The last part of her viewpoint, "All lessons in life will be repeated until learned," has always stuck with me. It's quite similar to how we must respect musculoskeletal dysfunction. If we ignore it, it will return in another form or a different region of the body or maybe even as internal (visceral) dysfunction. Dysfunction breeds dysfunction, so take action and determine the steps necessary to open the path toward wellness and healing.

Movement is medicine. It is more powerful than any pain reliever. Most musculoskeletal pain is of an ischemic nature. Skeletal joints are reliant upon movement for joint mobility and nutrition. Soft tissues (muscles, fascia, ligaments, and nerves) are dependent on movement for tissue gliding and local nutrition. Reduced nutrition impairs vascular and neural flow, leading to cellular changes that increase the risk for tissue overload. Movement restrictions are a top priority for restoring optimal function. Limited movement restricts the vital elements necessary for optimal function of musculoskeletal joints and tissues. Restoring motion requires skilled movement to build up natural movement patterns and tissue challenges to break down restrictions caused by pain-related behaviors and tissue overload.

We often fail to realize the nervous system is constantly dampening signals that could result in pain. It constantly measures whether information from the tissue is significant enough to warrant a response to impaired tension or dysfunctional movement. As long as a structural limit is compensated for by altered function in a nearby segment or adapted by a change in tension from a supportive loop, there is no pain. This compensation is driven by our task-oriented nervous system. Unfortunately, the part of the nervous system responsible for the movement system achieves maturity in the teenage years. I'm sad to report that your nervous system behaves like a teenager when it comes to the movement system. It rarely stops activity due to a limit or dysfunction, and it's very resistant to change, even if it's for the better. Instead, the nervous system will cause the musculoskeletal chain and myofascial loops to adapt and compensate with awkward movement or adverse tension, which can lead to tissue overload. Once a threshold is reached where movement and tissue nutrition are compromised, then pain becomes a signal of tissue overload.

How we reach this threshold is dependent upon how the brain responds to other factors. Sometimes, certain stressors or lifestyle factors can create a sensitivity or reduced pain threshold, thus making onset of pain more likely. The intricate relationship between wellness and healing is our true defense against musculoskeletal pain. Not everyone with structural deficits or functional imbalances develops pain. The determining factor is not always tissue function in terms of strength, stability, and mobility. Oftentimes, we must consider the overall health of our body and mind to get back on track after an injury or in the presence of persistent pain.

Structural deficits of musculoskeletal tissue are normal and unpreventable. Function of the entire neuromusculoskeletal system is the key to restoring balance and triggering healing, but it takes a wholesome approach.

5

TANGLED, NOT BROKEN

*Balance is not something you
find, it's something you create.*
—JANA KINGSFORD

Musculoskeletal pain is caused by dysfunction, not disease. Instead of pathology, it involves a pathway of dysfunction due to tissue overload related to poor nutrition and loss of tissue alliance. Impaired tissue alliance occurs when tension is no longer sufficient to maintain stability and mobility of the movement system. This intricate system involves more than three hundred muscle groups and an even greater number of joints that must maintain optimal tension and nutrition to remain healthy. Eventually, some segments or pathways will develop tissue changes that impair function or restrict freedom of movement that impairs tissue nutrition, essentially causing the myofascial loops to become tangled. The movement system remains capable despite dysfunction, but there are limits to its ability to adapt and compensate.

Each fiber of the muscular system is wrapped in fascia,

forming paths of myofascial tension that must be able to glide freely both within their series and among the neighboring myofascial loops. A movement limit or loading imbalance causes a loss of friction-free gliding, thus making fascial connections denser and stiffer as local nutrition and tissue mobility become restricted. With the immense integration of the fascial layers throughout the movement system, there is

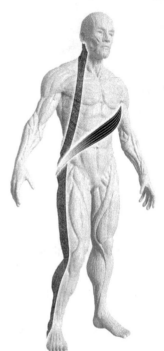

no chance for restrictions to occur in an isolated fashion. The task-driven nervous system simply increases the tension at neighboring or adjacent myofascial loops to compensate for the tangled pathways. This natural process of compensations allows us to still complete tasks despite movement dysfunctions. Yet it can lead to the tangled loops of tension, creating tissue overload particularly at links of the musculoskeletal chain, which may already have some degenerated or restricted structures.

Oftentimes I will get the question, "Why can't I just heal and be done with this problem?" The reality is that tissue has a memory. In a practical sense, we have all experienced tissue memory while performing a practiced skill or recalling a significant trauma. Yes, it involves neural drive and episodic memory but there must be something more on a local or peripheral level. In an editorial on fascial

Illustration of tangled myofascial loop: dysfunction along the paths of myofascial loop will cause an imbalance of myofascial tension, leading to compensatory movement strategies and increased potential for tissue overload.

science and clinical applications, Dr. Tozzi explains the basis for tissue memory. "Thus, since fascia appears to be organized in tensile myofascial bands, that comprise a single continuous structure, the repercussion of an intra-fascial restriction may be body-wide, and may potentially create stress on any structures enveloped by, or connected to, fascia. Dysfunctional memory might therefore be imprinted by the development of fibrous infiltration and cross links between collagen fibers at the nodal points of fascial bands, together with a progressive loss of elastic properties." (Tozzi 2014). Whether it's a neural pattern or tissue preference, compensatory movement strategies rarely correct themselves. Once a myofascial loop becomes tangled with trigger points and functional imbalances (WIS), it doesn't return entirely to normal. Yes, it can heal, but that simply means some level of balance is restored. The tangles remain embedded to some degree within the myofascial loop, making it predisposed to dysfunction whenever some other challenge or imbalance occurs. This is why problems can easily become recurrent along a tangled myofascial loop. It's not broken; it's just tangled, making it more susceptible to restricted movement or impaired loading.

Susan is a forty-two-year-old teacher with a long history of recurrent back and neck pain. She recently took a fall while hiking along rough terrain in the Alaskan wilderness. She recovered quickly but soon developed pain along the back of her thigh and leg. It seemed that she was taking a turn for the worse when she began to experience diffuse back and neck pain with vague tingling along both lower extremities. Her symptoms became widespread and debilitating, causing her to fear that the fall had caused serious damage. She struggled to manage even simple tasks at work, and any attempt to resume exercise resulted in diffuse pain in her hip and opposite shoulder. Even her students began to ask if she was all right since she had developed a noticeable limp and guarded movements. She decided it was time to ask her doctor to order an MRI. Soon after, she discovered the cause of her pain was due to multiple levels of degeneration in the spinal joints and discs, similar to this illustration:

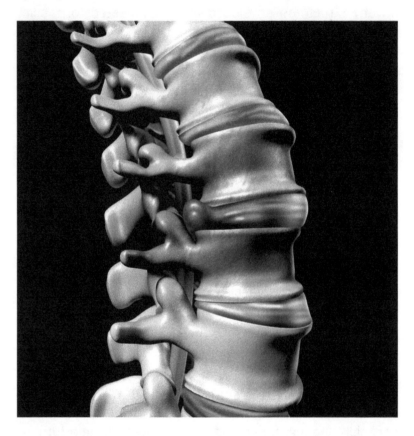

Susan was determined to avoid surgery, so she was offered a prescription for pain medications and referred to pain management for an epidural steroid injection. After her condition failed to improve, she began trying alternative treatment options. The outcome was variable; sometimes she felt better after chiropractic or massage, but the symptoms returned with any attempt to resume normal activity.

She was desperate and began to consider the possibility of surgery. Yet she was encouraged by a friend to try a different approach, since she experienced recovery with physical therapy. When I first met Susan, she was really on edge. She couldn't sustain any posture for prolonged periods due to pain, and she was very concerned about her ability to continue working. She didn't think her fall was significant enough to cause such excruciating pain, but her back and neck pain had never been this irritable. During the course of a thorough history and movement analysis, it became clear that she was dealing with a musculoskeletal dysfunction. She had limited movement at multiple links in the chain and significant regions of weakness and stiffness in the frontal myofascial loop. These restrictions were significant enough to cause her to walk as though she was being pulled in one direction, which caused her to lean sideways and load unevenly during each step.

After the evaluation, she asked me to review the MRI images, about which she said, "It shows how my spine is so messed up." Since I'm not an expert on imaging, I asked Susan, "How long do you think these changes took to occur?" She looked at the degenerative changes on the image that showed bone spurs and discs protrusions, then stated the obvious, "A long time." Now we were getting somewhere.

Susan easily recognized the structural changes on imaging as age-related adaptations. My goal was to help her understand that pain is more related to function than structure. I explained that since her spine has lived with loading for more than forty years and much of that time was spent without pain, then some other factor must be causing pain. We discussed how structural changes occur naturally due to age and loading. There was definitely reason to celebrate that the MRI failed to show any pathology; instead it simply showed age-related signs of degeneration. I explained the structural problems on her MRI have likely been there for years; "So why is it a problem now?" Her spine was not broken or damaged; it was simply showing signs of normal wear and tear. Since her pain was not an indication of damage, there must be a functional imbalance that is resulting in tissue overload. "We can't change the structure, but do you think it's possible for you to improve strength and movement?" The relief on her face was genuine as she realized that pain relief did not require us to fix the MRI.

For years, Susan had lived with variable patterns of symptoms despite the constant presence of these structural deficits. The problem was not solely due to structural changes; instead, it was more related to the functional limits within the musculoskeletal chain. Her movement showed obvious signs of myofascial restrictions disrupting the complex balance of tissue nutrition and mobility. Essentially, her tissue alliance was distorted by tangles in the myofascial loops, which was causing tissue overload at the degenerated segments of the spine. Unravelling these tangles would require healing movement to improve mobility and strength throughout the entire chain. Once we addressed the dysfunctional segments to restore balance of tissue alliance, "she could return to her previously dysfunctional self." We are all tangled to some degree; finding a balance between function and structure allows us to restore tissue alliance and live with less pain.

The health of the musculoskeletal system is solely dependent upon maintaining a balance between tissue loading and nutrition. Tissue nutrition is dependent upon variable movement to allow optimal blood and neural flow throughout the entire musculoskeletal chain. Since the neurovascular system is contained within the muscle and fascial layers, there is potential for compromise of tissue nutrition in the presence of functional imbalance (WIS). Tissue loading is altered as the nervous system adapts movement strategies to compensate for an imbalance of myofascial tension. This imbalance can spread and lead to tissue overload (MOD) as the myofascial loops attempt to compensate. The degenerated structures that were previously benign or nonpainful will experience excessive load and stress by the tangled myofascial loop, hence triggering ischemia (impaired tissue nutrition), which leads to a cycle of pain and inflammation.

Tissue loading is optimal when a tension state is present during movement. Tension is derived from myofascial loops aligned in a supportive fashion from the head to heel. Tangles in one or more pathways can result in compression compensating for the lack of tension. Typically, our musculoskeletal system can withstand these alterations in support if the tissue nutrition remains sufficient, but it can be a challenge when the entire loop is affected. If a tension imbalance occurs along the oblique myofascial loop, it may trigger tissue overload at the hip and opposite shoulder since this loop crosses the midline of the trunk. As the nervous system continues to demand tension from the weakened segments, stiffness begins to develop throughout other regions of the myofascial loop. Instead of developing tension in response to movement and loading, a compressive state may develop as other myofascial loops compensate for the imbalance. This is why it's so common for patients to present with more than just one complaint. A tangled myofascial loop will often result in hip and shoulder pain or back and neck pain.

The effects of this tension imbalance can impact any region along the chain affected by the tangled loop. This is where diagnosis of pain is extremely difficult, frustrating both the patient and provider. Since tissue overload may occur anywhere along the tangled route, there is little value in focusing only at the painful site. As tissue overload persists, the impaired flow of blood (ischemia) and nerve conduction increases the risk for pain and inflammation.

The degenerated or weakened structures are the first to experience pain. However, muscles and fascia along the tangled path can cause both local and referred pain. The only option to achieve healing is to restore movement and untangle the myofascial restrictions to restore optimal tissue loading throughout the entire chain.

The most important distinction about common musculoskeletal conditions is pain does not equal harm. Pain is not a sign of tissue damage; it's merely a loss of tissue alliance. More importantly, pain is not solely related to findings of degeneration on imaging. Nor is the painful site the same as the problem area. Our body follows a downward spiral of degeneration once growth and development slow in early adulthood. Nearly every tissue within the musculoskeletal system is in a constant state of breakdown and buildup. This is not necessarily a bad predicament, but it's a fact that we must prepare our movement system for the changes that occur throughout life. Maintaining optimal function of the chain through variable movement and three-dimensional strength creates a supportive tissue alliance that allows function to augment structure in a way that balances tissue loading. Maintaining tissue mobility and nutrition are the keys to defending against degeneration and dysfunction (Daneshmandi 2017).

Grace is a thirty-three-year-old bartender with recent onset of dizziness and vertigo. She awoke one morning with a severe headache, which quickly progressed to dizziness and vertigo. Her symptoms were so sudden and severe that she feared it was a serious pathology. After multiple visits to specialists and repeated trials of medication, she became frustrated with the endless tests and lack of answers. Plus, she still could not return to work due to the frequent bouts of vertigo. She did her own research on the web and came up with a regiment of exercises, but the progress was slow. Yet it was obvious that movement was a far better prescription than any other treatment thus far.

During our initial consult, Grace made it clear that she simply wanted some exercises to help resolve the dizzy problem. To her disappointment, I dragged her through a comprehensive evaluation and history, which uncovered some interesting indicators of dysfunction. First, she had a recurrent pattern of neck pain and headaches with symptoms often causing her to self-manipulate her neck. Next, she admitted that the prone position (on the belly) was her preferred sleeping position. Lastly, she developed her symptoms soon after an upper respiratory infection (flu-like symptoms). She described patterns of dizziness that made it nearly impossible to focus on a task while moving. She exclaimed, "I can pour a beer from the tap, but I can't carry it to the counter without fear of the room spinning." Her pattern of symptoms and onset made it quite clear that the musculoskeletal chain was definitely involved in the onset of dizziness. Before I could move on to some detailed testing, Grace had a few more symptoms to share. "I always get muscle spasms and tightness in the upper back after a day at work." I asked how she manages this problem. "I just spend ten to fifteen minutes rolling it out with a foam roller." After a bit of prodding, she admitted that it only helped temporarily. Next, she offered that she had a history of lower extremity sprains. In fact, she had a serious sprain of her ankle and midfoot about two years ago but failed to address it simply due to a busy schedule and lack of insurance. Eventually, her detailed history illustrated how functional limits of the myofascial loops could distort position sense and alter movement awareness. On their own, it's unlikely that these behaviors and patterns of functional limitations would be significant enough to cause vertigo and dizziness. But the combined influence of multiple dysfunctions throughout the chain and tangled myofascial loops could easily lead to a complex musculoskeletal condition.

In order to fully understand musculoskeletal dysfunction, it's necessary to appreciate two interdependent and interrelated elements of the musculoskeletal system. Both the structure and function of the tissue contribute directly to tissue alliance. Essentially, tissue alliance affords homeostasis and equilibrium within the musculoskeletal system, whereby movement is supported for the sake of withstanding loads. It would be shortsighted to diagnose a digestive problem without considering the structure and function of the entire GI system. Similar to other body systems, the musculoskeletal system has a dual purpose: movement and response to loading. Assessing only the structural elements while ignoring the potential for functional barriers is beyond shortsighted. Tissue alliance relies upon a balance of compression and tension throughout the chain to allow movement and load bearing. Disruption of this alliance often involves both structural and functional problems. The beauty of the movement system is its ability to allow gains in function to restore tissue alliance and compensate for structural deficits.

Getting all tangled up is typically the reason function fails to compensate for structure. The musculoskeletal system is not perfect; there are limits to what deficits and shortcomings can be overcome. Recent advances in imaging offer medical specialists the ability to identify even the slightest structural lesions and degenerative changes in the musculoskeletal chain. However, the musculoskeletal system is designed to withstand normal wear and tear. Structural degeneration involving ligament sprains, muscle strains and tears, disc herniations, cartilage breakdown, and nerve irritations are not the sole cause of pain; instead, they are simply the site of potential tissue overload due to a loss of tissue alliance. Remember, freedom of movement and response to loading are essential to health of the musculoskeletal system. Disruption of this finite balance between structure and function will result in some form of compensatory movement and altered tension patterns.

Impaired tissue alliance will often result in compensatory changes in function or tissue overload of weakened structures. Either outcome may set the stage for pain and inflammation. Let's consider how a simple weakness in the hip rotator muscles can affect tissue alliance of the entire musculoskeletal chain. Hip rotation weakness is a significant predictor for lower extremity injuries among adult women (Verrelst 2018). Like other muscles of the oblique myofascial loop, the gluteal muscle group plays an important role in both structure and function of the entire movement chain. The rotator cuff of the hip improves structural integrity of the hip by creating compressive forces that align the hip joint for smooth gliding during movement. Passive tension compresses the femoral head in a central location, giving the hip stability for loading activities. Active tension generates forces necessary to power the hip and balance movement. Essentially, the rotator cuff, whether at the hip or shoulder, is the perfect example of a mobile stabilizer. All segments of the musculoskeletal chain are important but not equal. Impaired function (WIS) at a mobile stabilizer requires far more force from other segments to compensate for the loss of tissue alliance. Not only due to the important role of rotation to allow movement throughout the chain but also because the adjacent myofascial loops are less effective at controlling rotation, and more effort is required to respond to loading outside their vector of force. This is typically how compensatory changes in function can cause painful movement in the absence of degeneration. Oftentimes, a segment critical to stability and mobility of the region becomes weak or unstable, which challenges our nervous system to adopt compensatory movement patterns to stay on task.

It's important to realize life goes on and tasks must be completed by our nervous system despite functional imbalances. Typically, the nervous system maintains tissue alliance without our knowledge through minor alterations in myofascial tension or shifting more compression onto structural segments through altered movement patterns. The nervous system has limited options for compensation to adapt to or overcome dysfunction. It simply does the least and hopes for the best. Sometimes it gets it right, especially if the movement system is healthy and wellness is sufficient to support healing. It's rare for a client to complain of the cause of their pain; many don't recognize that gluteal weakness led to their knee pain or back injury. They fail to notice that the job of the butt muscles has been overtaken by the back muscles. Just like it takes two average workers to replace one good worker, the same is true with a loss of tissue alliance. Nearby and adjacent muscles have to work harder to pick up the slack for functional imbalances. In a study comparing subjects during a lifting task, altered muscle patterns and impaired movement were present among those suffering from low back pain (LBP). LBP patients experienced 26 percent greater spine compression and 75 percent greater lateral shear (normalized to moment) than the asymptomatic group during the controlled exertions. The increased spine loading resulted from muscle coactivation and improper alignment (Marras 2002).

Most people with musculoskeletal pain have no idea their symptoms are related to a compensatory movement strategy with altered patterns of myofascial tension. In other words, they don't realize that pain is due to a loss of tissue alliance. For those with a combination of spinal pain and hip or shoulder pain, it becomes obvious early in the examination that their stability muscles have taken on a dual role as postural support and force production. For instance, the trunk muscles are not adequately suited to control rotation at the hip or shoulder, so there is a poorly coordinated alliance among nearby myofascial loops to take on dual roles as primary movers and mobile stabilizers. Multitasking is not optimal for our brain or our body. Eventually, compensatory patterns of myofascial tension and altered movement strategies will lead to tissue overload. Still, the tissue overload is usually far removed from the dysfunctional segments or pathways, which makes it pointless to only look at the painful site (Nakashima 2015).

Tissue overload is the endgame for loss of tissue alliance. Compensatory movement strategies lead to misalignment of rotation centers (hip/shoulder/ankle) where decentralization of the joint causes tissue overload of cartilage and ligaments. The vast number of nerves traveling within the muscle chain become susceptible to irritation and impingement due to the loss of balanced movement and impaired tissue nutrition. Whether or not the tissue overload leads to musculoskeletal pain is primarily dependent upon the level of wellness and healing potential. Our musculoskeletal chain is constantly striving to maintain tissue alliance, which is a very good reason to live to be well and move to heal.

A quick anatomy lesson is useful to appreciate the role of different tissues in musculoskeletal dysfunction. Cartilage is avascular once it is mature in the young adult, thus leaving it predisposed to degeneration from normal use. Although cartilage is considered a shock absorber, it is immensely dependent on the myofascial loops for withstanding loads. Positive findings on imaging showing tears in cartilage may simply be age-appropriate, physiological adaptations to tissue loading. Even in the case of degenerative tears, the myofascial loops can compensate for the reduced load tolerance of cartilage.

If it's a traumatic tear, such as an acute lesion of the labrum or meniscus, then functional recovery may be more difficult in the short term. Of course, the joint has limited ability to self-repair cartilage damage, but the reality is joint loading is not borne alone by cartilage. Myofascial tension is a far better shock absorber than cartilage, but it takes time to build sufficient strength and control to restore joint stability.

The spinal disc has similar characteristics to cartilage and ligaments, thus allowing it to respond with tension and compression during loading. Every activity causes spinal loading to some degree. Positive findings on imaging showing disc lesions such as herniation, bulging, and protrusion are typical of all adult spines regardless of whether pain is present or not (Brinjikji 2015). Discs are meant to bulge, just like the tire on your car. Many people will fall victim to the disease-based diagnosis, "You've got a slipped disc," "Your discs are herniated and flattened," "This is the worse spine I've ever seen," or "You are practically bone on bone." Yet these types of degenerative findings occur over the course of years, whereby the musculoskeletal system is able to compensate and adapt with changes in tissue function to balance loading. It's not the structure that needs to be repaired; it's the function that must be improved to restore tissue alliance.

Nerves are conduits of information via a chemical and conductive route that provide information to the nervous system and afford a path to effect changes in myofascial tension and joint movement. Positive findings on imaging often indicate structural deficits as the likely cause of nerve impingement. Oftentimes the nerve will be inflamed or enlarged at the impingement site, created by a bone spur or disc bulge. The reality is that nerves need movement, but surgical removal of the structural deficit often fails to restore movement. So what gives? Nerve mobility is dependent upon the balance of function throughout the entire pathway of the nerve, which is far more dependent on myofascial function than bony structures. Keep in mind that the nerves travel a far greater distance as vessels embedded in the muscles and fascia than along their path near bones and discs. Nerves do not need to be surgically released; they simply need to glide freely throughout the chain and loops.

Reaching an age of maturity often means settling into a sedentary lifestyle with a steady career path, which leads to more seat time and less physical activity. This settling down is coupled with tissue changes in the aging body that lean more toward functional imbalances. Movement is important as we age, but it becomes vital for those over age twenty-five. Sarcopenia is an example of tissue being on the clock. As we age, our collagen adapts and degenerates, causing involuntary loss of muscle mass, reduced strength, and loss of function. Sarcopenia can cause approximately 3–8 percent decrease of muscle mass per decade after the age of twenty-five. A similar effect occurs in aging cartilage as reduced depth and strength of cartilage impacts joint stiffness and loading (Mosher 2004). The effects are even more striking for the less active. Let's face it, the movement system needs variable activity to nourish the musculoskeletal chain and myofascial loops to defend against the natural, physiological changes caused by aging and reduced activity. Less movement as we age results in muscle weakness and joint stiffness, which reduces our ability to withstand loading. Rather than decreasing activity or becoming more sedentary with age, it's important to take on new activity and enjoy variable movements to challenge the movement system to become more mobile, stabile, and stronger.

Musculoskeletal pain is a direct result of impaired tissue alliance whereby restrictions in movement and nutrition directly impact the function of muscles, joints, and nerves.

It's a guaranteed human experience due to the fact that life is tissue loading. What a tangled web we weave! Life leads to tangles in the musculoskeletal system. There's no need to treat musculoskeletal conditions as a disease. There's no pill that can restore function. There's no need to fix the MRI. Choosing the fix only increases the risk of further dysfunction and disability. Medical management of musculoskeletal pain ignores the important role of tissue alliance. Instead, the over-reliance on imaging, drugs, and surgery is a warped and disastrous approach to a problem that should be addressed with wellness and healing. When it comes to addressing the functional imbalances of musculoskeletal dysfunction, movement is the best treatment option for recovery. Get moving and get strong to restore tissue alliance and prevent the detrimental effects of tissue overload.

PAIN IS A NATURAL
PART OF HEALING

Although the world is full of suffering,
it is full also of the overcoming of it.
—HELEN KELLER

The real question welling up to the surface as I evaluate clients with musculoskeletal pain is a big, bold "Why do I hurt?" It's a valid question when we continue to hear conflicting answers from health care providers and the scientific literature. I did my best to listen with unbiased interest during a recent graduate student presentation on the topic of soft tissue healing. It was a tongue-in-cheek reminder of how the medical system focuses on structural patterns of tissue repair but completely ignores functional recovery. Unfortunately, I was too quick to share this reality with the presenter, but it only served to confuse and distract the audience. Sometimes I wonder if I'm just a stranger on a strange planet. I can't be the only one who realizes musculoskeletal dysfunction is not solely defined by structural changes, nor is healing resigned only to tissue repair.

In order to understand musculoskeletal pain, there has to be some consideration of the purpose of pain. Remember, when it comes to musculoskeletal dysfunction, pain is more a sign of an imbalance rather than a sign of damage. There are three distinct phases of healing that are not fully understood, especially since pain may be present at any point in the process. Healing from a musculoskeletal condition is likened to a desert storm. It's unpredictable, but once it starts, there's no stopping it. The phases of tissue healing involve defense, repair, and recovery.

Tissue defense may be triggered by injury or imbalance. Tissue alliance can no longer support loading, which compromises tissue nutrition and leads to tissue overload. The nervous system goes on the defense due to the ischemic and inflammatory response as the tissue is shielded from further loading. As other segments accept additional loading and myofascial tension becomes altered, we near the point where tissue overload may breach the threshold for triggering pain. Most of us have one or more segments in the chain hovering in this defensive phase, whereby the condition remains subthreshold as the nervous system attempts to alter the tension and movement to maintain some balance. This is the ticking time bomb nature of musculoskeletal dysfunction. What keeps it from igniting is the state of wellness. Keeping well is our best option to improve tissue defense and resolve musculoskeletal pain.

Once defense fails to properly compensate for an imbalance or injury, there is a cascade of events that lead to tissue repair. How much and how long is dependent upon factors such as genetics, age, lifestyle, and nutrition. During tissue repair, inflammation drives cells to the tissue with the potential to either heal or further inflame the region. This is what makes inflammation a necessary but also potentially damaging component of repair. If the dependent factors are well suited for healing, then the inflammation is resolved overtime as the cells turn over and blood flow is restored. Otherwise the inflammation becomes persistent and is either maintained at a low boil or boils over. Inflammation tends to set the stage for more persistent or severe pain, causing stark limits of tissue nutrition and movement. Pain due to inflammation has a couple of obvious indicators. It tends to get easily wound up, and it can make even normal movements painful.

This is a difficult turn of events since movement is the only method to restore tissue nutrition and quell the inflammation. Of course, the inflammatory cycle could be interrupted with medication, but it must be combined with movement; otherwise there's no hope in moving forward to the final phase of healing.

The last phase of healing, which is often ignored, is tissue recovery. Recovery of muscle activation and restoration of normal movement patterns is critical to restoring balance of tissue alliance. Recall that during the initial phase of healing, there is an automatic shielding of the dysfunctional segments and paths from further loading. This creates a redundant compensatory pattern with multiple segments of tissue overload due to the presence of WIS throughout the chains and loops. Segments will become stiff or unstable, causing improper alignment and decentralization of joint surfaces. Myofascial tension will either be delayed in activation or altogether silent during loading. Reactivating myofascial tension and correcting joint alignment requires skilled movement and controlled loading to restore tissue alliance. Otherwise the nervous system will revert back to shielding the dysfunctional segments. Compensatory movement patterns can only be corrected by retraining balanced joint alignment and myofascial tension in a variety of positions to retrain stability and restore mobility in all three dimensions of movement. Full recovery is dependent upon skilled movement and controlled loading to achieve optimal function of the movement system.

7

*Healing is a matter of time, but it is
sometimes also a matter of opportunity.*
—HIPPOCRATES

Many times, clients will attempt to see their pain through
the same blinders used by the medical fix approach, hoping their problem and pain are one and the same. The
reality is that you can't always trust pain. Tissue does not
have a direct path to the brain to signal an imbalance.
Instead, there are overlapping channels and varying influ-
ences that tend to alter the region and intensity of the
symptoms. The tissue bluff is evident in areas that are
either chronically painful or close (proximal) to the trunk.
Essentially if a region has been painful for some time, the
nervous system will adapt to make those symptoms more
relevant and readily accessible. It's a simple feature of
adaptation both at the site of pain and within the nervous
system to protect the painful region. Areas close to the
trunk like the hip, shoulder, and spine lack detailed maps

within the nervous system, making the pain site a poor indicator of the problem area.

Myofascial pain can involve local and referred pain. Local pain occurs at the site of the tissue problem. If you hit your thumb with a hammer, then the site of the problem (bum thumb) is also the site of the pain. As time passes, symptoms may extend to the wrist and entire hand. Part of this expansion of the pain area is a protective response by the nervous system designed to limit further damage. The other aspect of referred pain involves impaired tissue nutrition and inflammation. Referred pain is the hallmark feature of chronic musculoskeletal conditions. Prolonged periods of tissue overload lead to a neural shielding of the region whereby the nervous system reduces muscle activation and alters movement patterns to protect the tissue. This creates a mild form of neural or cortical neglect where the lack of activation and altered motion leads to impaired tissue nutrition (ischemia). Eventually, these neglected segments will develop tissue restrictions, such as trigger points and fascial restrictions, which are prone to inflammation with tissue overload. Depending on the irritability of trigger points, pain can refer well beyond the actual site of the problem.

Chronic pain has the potential to develop referred pain. Essentially, the pain may extend well beyond the painful region. Contrary to the disease framework, more pain is not a result of more damage. Instead, referred pain is caused by the multifactorial nature of pain. Basically, once other systems become involved in the pain process, there is a combination of factors that contribute to the persistent painful state. The pain is no longer due solely to mechanical problems such as functional imbalance and tissue overload. Chemical changes such as inflammation both at the site of the problem and within the terminal points of the nervous system influence the pain map. This is accompanied by changes in the attitude and response to pain, better known as psychosocial and emotional behaviors, which influence the pain process. Lastly, general health and wellness affect the degree and pattern of symptoms. The multifactorial pain map can be challenging to navigate since it takes more than one approach to achieve pain relief.

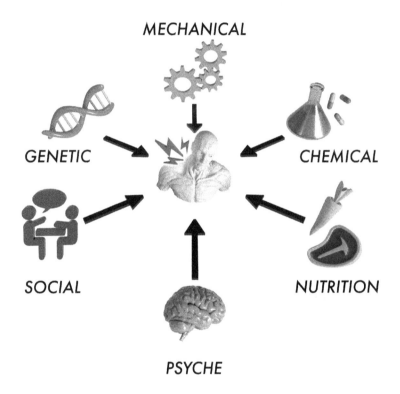

Unfortunately, exposing the tissue bluff is not a simple cause-effect scenario. Simply treating the cause may not resolve pain; in fact, it may worsen symptoms as the nervous system interprets any input as an insult. The presence of referred pain requires a gradual change in all factors contributing to the pain process to create subtle changes that create a healing environment. It requires an individualized approach to improve tissue alliance throughout the entire chain and enhance the Wellness SAFE. No pill or procedure can alter the pain process sufficiently to resolve referred pain. Changing the pattern of overmedicalization of musculoskeletal pain requires us to recognize pain as a sign of impairment of movement, warranting an approach that is geared toward healing a dysfunction rather than fixing a disease.

Tissue bluff and referred pain are unique concepts that truly define musculoskeletal conditions as dysfunctions rather than disease. Basically, you can't trust the location of pain and the problem to be one and the same. This complex nature of pain was made clear by my recent encounter with a local pilot. Phillip owns a well-drilling operation, and he recently came across my property while flying with his wife. He was impressed by our cabin overlooking the river and wanted to take a closer look. He stopped by unannounced with hopes of getting a better look at our view of the river. Since we live remotely in Willow, I was a bit suspicious, but I gave him the benefit of doubt. He explained that he was recently married, and he was taking his bride on a sightseeing flight along the range when he came across our picturesque view. "I just couldn't stop doing flyovers. It was so beautiful from above." I welcomed him to take a look around to see the view from ground level. As soon as he stepped out of the truck, I noticed he was suffering from pain. He took short strides and shifted his weight as though he was avoiding loading on the heel of his right foot. I didn't want to mettle, so I gave him a tour of the property and shared some stories about our Alaskan experience. After watching the river from the cliff behind our home, Phil asked about my plans for the property. I explained that we are still in the early stages, but my dream was to build a wellness retreat for clients and caregivers. "Are you a doctor?" he asked.

I explained, "Yes, I'm a doctor of physical therapy." And so the story began as he started to relate his personal story of struggling with chronic pain.

Phillip is fifty-five years old and has been struggling with heel pain for the past few months. Recently, it's gotten so bad that he can barely stand for more than a few minutes and walking without shoes is nearly impossible. His wife finally convinced him to go to the doctor. After wasting more time in the lobby than in the exam room (according to Phil's description), the doctor diagnosed his symptoms as plantar fasciitis and prescribed an anti-inflammatory. When I asked Phil if this approach was helpful, he immediately replied, "Zilch. Notta."

I asked him, "Well, how long have you had LBP?"

Without hesitation, he said, "Forever." He further explained, "No big deal. Nearly all the men in my line of work have to deal with LBP." He admitted he recently reduced field work due to the number of administrative tasks, which has resulted in most of his day being spent sitting at the desk. Over the past few months, he developed severe right heel pain, making it extremely difficult to exercise or walk for any distance. As the story covered more detail, it became clear that his problem was not located at the ankle or foot. Yes, his pain was at the heel, but the problem was definitely farther up the chain.

Chronic musculoskeletal pain is rarely a sign of injury or tissue damage. For instance, common complaints of heel pain typically associated with plantar fasciitis are more often due to overload of the posterior myofascial loop. The pain may be evident at the heel, but the real problem (WIS) is farther up the chain at the hip or back. Since most musculoskeletal pain is referred to an area far removed from the problem, it's more relevant to consider referred pain as a sign of tissue loading rather than tissue damage. Pain is a mode of communication our nervous system utilizes to call our attention to tissue overload (MOD). In this case, pain is no longer a threat; it's actually a challenge to make a change in how we load tissue. Our only option is to identify functional imbalances (WIS) and restore tissue alliance throughout the chain.

An example of a simple injury becoming a chronic pain problem is a ligament sprain. Ankle sprains are the most common lower extremity ligament injury. Although this region is poorly vascularized, it will heal with simple principles of rest, ice, compression, and elevation (RICE). But there's a reason this simple injury often leads to a chronic condition known as functional ankle instability (FAI). FAI is one of the most common musculoskeletal conditions, causing persistent ankle pain and poor balance with recurrent ankle sprains. The fact is that many people with a simple ankle sprain only achieve a limited recovery. The ankle ligament heals with tissue repair, but functional recovery is rarely achieved. This leaves the lower extremity subject to limited muscular support (weakness), uncontrolled motions (instability), and restricted motion (stiffness).

In order to achieve complete healing, RICE must be followed by MEAT (movement, exercise, activation, treatment) to fully recover tissue function. Tissue recovery must be accompanied by restoration of movement and stability of the chain and loops. Achieving improved tissue function by way of improving mobility, strength, and balance of tissue allows the movement system to easily compensate and adapt to structural limitations. As a general rule of thumb, improving function allows for existence of structural deficits without pain. Just like we can adapt to awkward positions or poorly balanced loads, our movement system is designed to accommodate structural imperfections. Yet it can't readily achieve functional recovery without some change in movement and loading to restore tissue alliance.

The osseous-ligamentous components of the musculo-skeletal system are designed to develop mass and integrity from youth to early adult. Sort of like the story of the three little pigs. Got to build a good house to prepare for the coming storms and wolves. The risks of sarcopenia combined with a sedentary lifestyle tilts the scale toward tissue breakdown. There is no chance in building new cartilage to unload the joint, nor can the disc repair itself to original structure. So what gives in those cases where heel pain resolves or LBP goes away and the structural problems remain? It's simply healing and restoring the function of the whole system rather than returning it to normal. Healing makes us whole again, but it does not return tissue back to its original state. The phases of healing progress from defense to recovery, how far and how fast it occurs, depends on the state of wellness and healing. Pain can occur at any phase either due to inflammation or tissue overload. Remember, it's possible to get stuck at any phase, so find a way to get moving and learn how to improve wellness so your body has the tools to heal.

Pain is never permanent.
—SAINT TERESA OF AVILA

Chronic musculoskeletal conditions like plantar fasciitis, rotator cuff tendonitis, and LBP don't mean you are sentenced to a lifetime of pain. Nothing stays the same when it comes to the musculoskeletal system. Tissue changes on a daily basis; it's either becoming more redundant in the painful pattern or it's turning the corner for healing. Failure to take action and make positive changes to improve wellness limits the ability of our nervous system to access the necessary elements for healing. Avoiding activity due to fear of pain or injury restricts movement and nutrition to tissue, thus impeding the inherent healing potential. In other words, the power is in your hands to turn chronic pain into a distant memory.

Chronic musculoskeletal pain sits under the guise of inflammation, such as an arthritis or tendonitis. Yet the reality is that just like other types of musculoskeletal pain, the tissue is not the issue. Many painful conditions are blamed on the presence of inflammation and a structural lesion such as a bone spur or tendon tear. Yet the inflammation is only present due to the tissue overload causing a restriction of normal movement and reduced blood flow. These restrictions combined trigger a cycle of pain and inflammation. This is tissue overload on a widespread scale where the nervous system has accepted that normal movement hurts. Simple movements ranging from getting out of a chair to carrying groceries can potentially provoke pain. As the nervous system awareness is primed for pain and movement patterns are altered, multiple segments become overloaded due to wide-ranging imbalances throughout the chain. Rather than a couple of weak or stiff segments, an entire region is functionally imbalanced. Pain can shift from one side to the other or affect a nearby region without warning. It can be frustrating and debilitating since most people tend to avoid activity, which only seems to worsen the problem.

Yet it's important to keep in mind that the painful or inflamed tissue is rarely the real problem. Many will choose to cling to the status quo explanation of chronic pain. They rely on some fix for the problems identified on MRI or some pill to remedy inflammation. Of course, this path has some serious drawbacks since there is no personal responsibility to make changes to improve wellness or take steps to activate healing potential. Failure to struggle is simply expecting others to clean up your mess. Remember, you are not broken, just tangled. Can you untie your own knot, or do you need someone to do it for you? It takes a bit of internal struggle to realize chronic pain has the ability to change if we are willing to change. Understanding that persistent pain is an imbalance in the load-bearing ability of the entire musculoskeletal system only means one thing. It's time to turn chronic into change. Get moving and get strong to restore optimal tissue loading and regain freedom of movement.

Most chronic conditions lack inflammation since the healing process has simply been aborted by the nervous system. The nervous system has a big job, and it must decide winners and losers on a daily basis. Some problems are simply too big to tackle. Failure to address imbalances (WIS) in the musculoskeletal chain leaves degenerated segments exposed to repeated cycles of tissue overload. The attempt to shield an area and avoid activation of movement for prolonged periods leads to a lack of tissue nutrition. Ischemia becomes the main culprit for chronic musculoskeletal pain as the nervous system reduces its output due to limited returns. Since loading can't be avoided altogether, there is less potential for healing, creating a cycle of tissue overload and reduced activity.

Coping with chronic pain is fraught with anxiety and fear since the main sign of success is focused on pain relief. This is where the mind shift must occur. Pain must be seen as an opportunity to restore movement and consider what you can achieve with less pain. Rather than recognizing hurt as harm, get excited to implement the changes that will move you closer to living with pain instead of painful living. Restoring tissue function and nutrition will not result in immediate change of symptoms. Chronic symptoms are slow to change, but pacing and consistency are the keys to success. Gradual changes to improve wellness will activate your healing potential. Healing will require frequent exercise to enhance mobility, stability, and strength throughout the musculoskeletal system. It's typical for pain to fluctuate throughout the healing process, but you can expect steady progress toward pain relief once balance is restored to tissue loading and nutrition.

It's the chain, not the image, that is causing the pain. So, contrary to what we have been told, the degenerated segment on imaging is simply a normal part of living. No need for repairing or replacing it with surgery, unless it involves acute trauma or pathology. Since chain replacements are currently not available, the only option is to trust in the healing potential of all tissue as small changes are made to restore tissue movement and nutrition. It's all about the function of the entire musculoskeletal system. If optimal tissue function is restored, then the musculoskeletal chain can easily compensate for structural restrictions, even those that look quite severe on imaging. In many musculoskeletal dysfunctions, a slight structural problem can become painful in the presence of major functional imbalances. Repeat occurrence or persistent pain does not indicate a lack of healing. Instead, it is an indication of limited or incomplete functional recovery leaving the musculoskeletal chain imbalanced and at risk. On the flip side, major structural lesions on imaging can be painless if the function of myofascial loops is optimal. So, if you want pain relief, you only have to look in the mirror.

Will is a fifty-three-year-old flight line supervisor. He has struggled with chronic LBP for decades that sometimes requires him to miss work or avoid certain activities. Like most people with LBP, he doesn't recall the exact onset, but he suspects it's related to years of competitive bodybuilding and labor-intensive work. Over the past couple years, his pain has become more persistent, with nearly any physical activity triggering symptoms. Plus, he has developed knee and shoulder pain, further aggravating his symptoms. He's tried working out at the gym and increasing his stretching routine, but nothing seems to help. Upon his first visit with a physician, he was shocked to hear that back surgery would be necessary. Yes, the MRI showed a flat disc and bone on bone at multiple segments in the spine, but he was reluctant to consider surgery as an option. He denied the referral for pain medications and instead asked for a referral to physical therapy. Soon after our first consult, Will was impressed with the chain approach demonstrating how one dysfunction leads to another. He was ready to make changes in his attitude toward pain and willing to slow things down to allow tissue to be moved and loaded within its capacity to heal. Will is living with pain, but he's living well. His back pain is minimal or nonexistent on some days. He is still working to restore knee mobility and shoulder strength, but he is on track to getting a life back he never thought possible.

This case illustrates how a health care consumer can make the right choices when trying to navigate the medical system. Rather than blindly following the referral trail from imaging to drugs and surgery, a health care consumer seeks the remedy that will restore function with minimal risks. Don't fall victim to the flawed practice of the medical model applying disease-based rules to non-life-threatening musculoskeletal impairments and dysfunctions. Be a smart health consumer rather than a compliant patient.

SOMETIMES YOU
NEED A GUIDE

> *You get in life what you have*
> *the courage to ask for.*
> —OPRAH WINFREY

I often get the following introduction during new client evaluations. "I just want you to fix my pain" or "My MRI shows_____
. No way therapy can fix it." I try to be comprehensive in outlining the two sides of musculoskeletal pain, structure and function. I've limited time to make my pitch for healing. It's like starring on *Shark Tank*. I try various angles to get my client's attention off the fix fantasy and back to the reality of healing. Once I have a client who is excited about their prospects with a renewed hope in healing, it's time to begin the journey. Healing requires a mind-set and attitude to move forward despite setbacks or pitfalls. You need a guide who will encourage you to build a healing environment rather than point you back to the fix.

Healing from a musculoskeletal dysfunction is not a complex endeavor. Healing potential is present within every well human. Sometimes we need a competent guide to help us gain access to this healing potential. A healing guide could be a licensed therapist (physical or occupational therapist) or some other movement expert with relevant knowledge and experience in the musculoskeletal chain and healing. Asking a guide for help with healing pain is a reasonable approach since it won't result in a pill or procedure. Instead, you must be willing to make lifestyle changes to reclaim wellness and adopt a balanced approach toward eliminating the barriers to healing.

As a health consumer, you should accept that musculo-skeletal pain is inevitable. If pain fails to resolve with time and changes in activity, then you owe it to yourself to seek help. If you fail to get competent treatment for a musculo-skeletal dysfunction, then it will only lead to more dysfunction, potentially causing a more complex pain syndrome, which often leads people back to square one: seeking a fix. A healing guide should be a licensed provider to ensure their training and competence is valid. You should seek out a provider who will listen to your entire story rather than just asking where the pain is. If they can explain how your pain is directly related to your history and make some sense out of the functional imbalances identified by a thorough exam, then you've got a keeper. Essentially, you should expect three questions to be answered by your healing guide:

- What are the primary causes of my pain?
- What can I do to get better?
- How will you help me heal?

Proper treatment of musculoskeletal pain should include a multifaceted approach such as manual therapy and motor control. Manual therapy includes treatments to break down tissue restrictions while encouraging movement and blood flow. Treatments such as dry needling, manipulation, and mobilization help untangle compensatory patterns of tissue overload. This must be combined with exercise and motor learning to build up balanced patterns of movement. This time-dependent process of break down and build up is a near perfect platform to launch your healing journey. However, there are always potential pitfalls and barriers that may delay healing or prevent full recovery. Typically, it's a lack of wellness that can limit the body's ability to make use of healing interventions. Oftentimes, it's more related to bad lifestyle habits that may limit tissue nutrition. Either way, choosing a guide to coach and mentor you toward healing is a critical step for avoiding the fix. Healing is a worthwhile venture to recover from musculoskeletal pain; you deserve a guide who will help you start and complete the journey.

10
RESTORING
TISSUE ALLIANCE

*Rather than painful movement, consider how
to restore confidence and joy in movement.*
—KEITH

If you are willing to accept pain as an opportunity, then this is
your chance to take action. Tired of bearing witness to pain
being mistreated or overmedicalized? It's time to choose a
path toward healing. Restoring tissue alliance is the safest
and most reliable route for complete healing and pain relief.
Tissue alliance is the essence of complex movements and
our ability to efficiently respond to loading throughout the entire movement system. It is equilibrium within the movement
system where mobility is buffered by stability and strength
is augmented by balance. It's a highly complex relationship
between structure and function to ensure tension is balanced and controlled. Restoring tissue alliance is a gradual
progression of skilled movement and controlled loading to
allow tissue recovery and remobilize, recentralize, and reload
the movement system.

- Recovery: safe and supportive positions and movements for unloading and unwinding.
- Remobilize: multidirectional (3D) movement to challenge stiff links.
- Recentralize: balance and stability to retrain position sense and movement awareness.
- Reload: strength and controlled loading throughout the musculoskeletal system.

Recovery (Unwind and Unload)

Realizing that pain is a sign of imbalance or an opportunity for change doesn't simply make it disappear. Rather than fear or avoidance, it's time to ensure pain works in your favor. Symptoms may be aggravated with a specific position or posture, which can give clues to which loop is tangled or which segment is overloaded. Or perhaps a more dynamic pattern is related to an intermittent cycle of pain. Whether symptoms occur with static postures or dynamic tasks, it's important to determine a direction or loading preference for recovery. Pain with static postures suggests that dynamic activity is the best way to unwind and recover. Pain with movement in specific directions warrants recovery in positions that release stress and unload. For instance, if walking is painful, then consider stationary cycling or reclined ball walks. If sitting is painful, try air squats and side shuffle to recover.

Choose a position or activity for recovery that is supportive, symmetric, and stable (SSS). Use the SSS principles to recover from prolonged postures, extended activity, or strenuous exercise. The recovery position or activity should be a chance to unwind and unload from the day's stress. It should require minimal effort and allow a neutral position for the entire musculoskeletal chain. Maintain this position or activity for at least six to eight minutes. Recovery offers a perfect opportunity to practice deep breathing to calm the nervous system. The right position or activity can help augment nutrition flow for hydrophilic structures like the disc and cartilage. These structures are often dehydrated due to prolonged, static postures or repetitive loading, especially with any significant tissue overload and degeneration.

Remobilize (Get Moving)
Every well human moves to heal. Regardless of how you want to get moving, any movement is better than none at all. The goal is to maintain aerobic exercise for fifteen to twenty minutes daily. For the sake of mobility, it's important to resume movement regardless of the pain state. Keep in mind that pacing is the first step toward the healing path. If you are familiar with running, then start with a walk/jog/run routine. For instance, during initial stages of the routine, it's best to ration exercise on a gradual scale of difficulty. Try the 3-2-1 scale: walk three minutes / jog two minutes / run one minute. Or if you prefer cycling, consider starting with a stationary cycle. Either way, it's important to feed the chain what it desires most—movement.

Regaining mobility at restricted segments or tight pathways requires skilled movements to resolve stiffness and balance tissue load. Skilled movements are the key to untangling myofascial loops and improving nutrition flow to degenerated tissues. When the musculoskeletal chain becomes overburdened with stiff joints, a pattern of awkward postures and impaired movement strategies will become the norm, while restricted gliding and impaired mobility within the myofascial loops often lead to tissue overload and reduced nutrition. Regaining mobility does not require aggressive stretching or challenging calisthenics. It requires keen attention to skilled movement to access the full range of motion throughout the musculoskeletal chain while challenging the myofascial loops in all three dimensions of mobility, with emphasis on speed and accuracy of movement patterns.

Each link of the musculoskeletal chain has a preferred stiffness when it is not repeatedly challenged by variability of movement across all three dimensions of mobility. For instance, the ball and socket joints will develop limits in the transverse plane, restricting rotation. The hip, shoulder, and ankle are prone to limited rotation, which impairs force transmission and shock absorption. While hinge joints, like the elbow and knee, tend to stiffen in the sagittal plane, which limits bending or flexion and extension. A similar pattern of stiffness exists in the spine, whereby the neck is prone to stiffen with rotation while the thorax lacks extension. Remobilization of the musculoskeletal chain must address the inherent stiffness at multiple links to normalize movement patterns and retrain positional awareness.

Myofascial restrictions occur in specific pathways along a particular myofascial loop. Oftentimes, the site of pain may offer clues to the direction, rather than the location, of the problem. For instance, pain along the anterior aspect of the shoulder may indicate stiff links along the sagittal (anterior) myofascial loop. It's important to treat the entire loop by activating tension along the opposing pathways (posterior) to resolve the weakness that often accompanies stiffness. Local treatments such as mobilization or manipulation to the fascial pathway can be used to restore gliding and local tissue mobility. Initially, it's important to avoid direct treatment to the painful region, since the nervous system may interpret any input as an insult. Instead, better results can be attained by mobilizing the fascial pathway above and below the painful site. Working around the pain rather than at the pain allows the respective loop to lengthen and restore optimal tension.

Tack and glide the myofascial paths. Rub and scrub around the pain. Massage and mobilize the entire region. It's more than just tight muscles or stiff fascia. Myofascial tension has a neural drive that's task oriented and load responsive. Once you determine the restricted myofascial loop, it's possible to influence it anywhere along the path of tension. A stiff path will be sore and dense due to the tissue changes caused by lack of tissue gliding and impaired nutrition. It's important to break down tissue restrictions in a slow, gradual manner. Start with tack and glide at two or three sites along the path and finish with a gentle massage or mobilization of the entire region.

Tack and glide involves gentle, focused pressure and progressive friction in all three directions. It's possible to use a semirigid tool (3TOOL) or reinforced knuckle, but the gliding motion must be maintained for two to three minutes. Sort of like trying to remove a grease spot, just be sure to stay on the dense spot rather than moving it around or sliding on the skin. Once the path has improved gliding, it's helpful to transition to rub and scrub. Don't just rub nearby areas until sore; instead, apply consistent pressure around the dense area to assist with lymphatic and nerve flow. After fifteen to thirty seconds, the area should become less dense, and tissue warmth should be increased. Tack and glide is the preferred method to break down tissue restrictions, so it takes some time and effort. Rub and scrub is a quick method for restoring good sensory input to a painful area. Always finish with a gentle massage of the entire muscle or mobilization of nearby joints to retrain normal movement boundaries. Restoring joint space and reducing myofascial stiffness requires movements that unravel the tangles caused by our daily life.

Recentralize (Get Stable)

What was really significant about Achilles's heel? In the legend, the heel was Achilles's one weak link, left unprotected when his mother dipped him into protective waters. Likewise, there are weak and vulnerable joints throughout the entire musculoskeletal chain. The human nervous system drives the musculoskeletal chain like a race car avoiding risky loads at every turn. It relies on the feedback from the intricate fascial network to stabilize joints and respond to loading in the nick of time. Joint stability is more than just a tight articular capsule. It requires balanced activation of myofascial loops to ensure smooth gliding of articular surfaces and proper alignment during loading. But it's not a perfect system; joint and myofascial restrictions can cause articular surfaces to be decentralized. Decentralization is common at ball-and-socket joints where congruity is an important factor in joint stability and nutrition. Essentially, a decentralized joint requires more effort, meaning more compression, for normal movement, which compromises the local tissue nutrition and leads to tissue overload.

Decentralization is not the same as subluxation or malalignment. It's a simple matter of the myofascial tension being imbalanced. All joints require support from the myofascial loops to create stability during movement and loading. Some joints rely upon form closure to achieve stability, while others rely more upon force closure. For instance, the hip is quite stable due to the congruent articular surfaces allowing the ball to be seated well within the socket, particularly in weightbearing situations (form closure). Whereas the shoulder, being the most mobile joint in the body, relies fully upon myofascial tension to maintain stability (force closure). This tension creates joint compression to seat the gliding joint surfaces into the optimal position. The presence of ball-and-socket joints at transitional junctions demonstrates our need to augment movement with stability. At the base of the skull, the first spinal joint involves the ball-and-socket joint of the occipital condyles resting upon the deep sockets of the atlas. Each end of the extremities has proximal and distal ball-and-socket joints. The shoulder and hip are both ball-and-socket joints designed for loading and mobility. The more distal joints, like the wrist and ankle, are designed for rotation and force transmission. All of these joints share a common fault: they go wherever tension pulls. These joints are very dependent upon balanced tension forces to maintain a centralized position of the convex member (ball) seated within the concave surface (socket). Impingement of tissue (cartilage, muscle, nerve) can occur when joint alignment is decentralized.

Balance and stability training are the best methods to restore a central position to joint surfaces. Begin training in a safe setting that allows you to achieve success after a couple attempts. Use the SSS principles to progress the training. Progress from a supportive position, like the supine position, to a half-kneeling posture. Start with a symmetric position where both limbs are in contact with the surface to a more asymmetric posture where you are supported by only one extremity. Lastly, the challenge can be increased by moving from a static position to incorporating dynamic movements to challenge your balance. Stability of posture and neutral joint position should be maintained throughout the training to retrain a central position. More advanced training can incorporate the use of balance training aids like a half foam roll, therapeutic ball, or balance board. During upright training scenarios, be sure to choose a safe setup where there is no risk of falling, such as a doorway or hallway.

Reload (Get Strong)

The ability to handle physiological loading is the ultimate goal of tissue recovery. The movement system is designed to perform motion and respond to loading. A gradual return to loading requires variable activity and resistive exercise. Routine exercise should include some body weight exercises to help reach your target heart rate. Tissue is loaded with all activity; the key is balancing the load along the entire chain rather than hinging or leveraging it at one segment. Proper tissue loading requires attention to position and effort. Keep it neutral and balanced with gradual increases of effort. Consider transitioning from isometric to isotonic to load the entire fascial loop in a neutral posture. The goal is to transition from safe, static loading of all myofascial loops, followed by more dynamic exercise involving the entire musculoskeletal chain.

Restoring tissue alliance puts your healing potential into action. It's an active process of integrating skilled movements and controlled loading to improve tissue mobility and nutrition, which untangles the myofascial restriction and restores balanced loading to the musculoskeletal chain.

Visit www.newak.com for detailed guidance and videos on restoring tissue alliance

AFTERWORD

The standard choices for treatment of musculoskeletal pain have become nothing more than empty promises by health business. Misleading ad campaigns and medical trends can't change reality or mold science to justify pills or procedures as reasonable options to resolve musculoskeletal pain. Whether it's the pain epidemic or opiate crisis, health business has been there through it all. The emphasis on treating musculoskeletal pain as a disease has ramped up the use of imaging, drug prescriptions, and surgery. Drug interventions with limited applications have become widespread approaches to encompass nearly every ache and pain, leading Americans to be labeled the world's largest drug consumer. The rush to use surgery instead of encouraging the time-tested benefit of wellness and healing has amounted to higher rates of disability and more costly health care.

The writing has been on the wall for far too long. All health care providers and pain sufferers should be ready to exit the theatrical stage of the overmedicalization of musculoskeletal pain. It's time to accept personal responsibility for a strong Wellness SAFE and optimal healing potential as the best hope for resolving musculoskeletal pain. It's time to realize the true nature and meaning of musculoskeletal pain. Pain is not a threat or danger; it's an opportunity—an opportunity to appreciate how our musculoskeletal system is trying to compensate for movement dysfunction and health impairments.

Be the brave soul who admits there is no quick fix for painful musculoskeletal conditions. Our movement system does not require a fix to achieve pain relief. The musculoskeletal system has the potential to heal. You simply have to access the healing potential that already exists. Every well human moves to heal. It's time to stop playing the disease-laden health care game with musculoskeletal health. It's a gamble where the prize is tainted with dependency and disability. The war on musculoskeletal pain can never be won by drugs and surgery. To overcome musculoskeletal pain, the struggle starts with individuals recognizing musculoskeletal pain is simply an opportunity to change—change that must be taken by the individual to regain wellness and utilize the power of corrective movements to trigger healing, thus restoring balance within the musculoskeletal system, which leads to natural pain relief. Never underestimate the ability of the well human to move toward healing. Healing and wellness are inseparable; we live to be well and move to heal. Believe in the power of wellness and healing. Believe in what your body is trying to tell you. You have the power to heal.

REFERENCES

Abdallah, C., and H. Geha. 2017. "Chronic pain and chronic stress: Two sides of the same coin?" *Chronic Stress* 1: 10.

Aguirre, J., A. Borgeat, M. Hasler, P. Bühler, JM Bonvini. 2016. "Clinical concentrations of morphine are cytotoxic on proliferating human fibroblasts in vitro." *European Journal of Anesthesiology* 33, no. 11: 832–839.

Bennett, M., J. Zeller, L. Rosenberg, J. McCann. 2003. "The effect of mirthful laughter on stress and natural killer cell activity." *RN Alternative Therapies* 9, no. 2: 38–43.

Brinjikji W, et al. 2015. "Systematic literature review of imaging features of spinal degeneration in asymptomatic populations." *AJNR Am J Neuroradiol* 36(4):811–6.

Buchman A, et al. 2010. Musculoskeletal Pain and Incident Disability in Community-Dwelling Elders. *Arthritis Care Res* (Hoboken) 62(9): 1287–1293.

Centers for Disease Control: "Wide-ranging Online Data for Epidemiologic Research"

Committee on Advancing Pain Research, Care, and Education Board on Health Sciences Policy. Relieving Pain in America: A Blueprint for Transforming Prevention, Care, Education, and Research

Connizzo BK, et al. 2014. "The detrimental effects of systemic Ibuprofen delivery on tendon healing are time-dependent." *Clin Orthop Relat Res* 472(8):2433–9

Daneshmandi H, et al. 2017. "Adverse Effects of Prolonged Sitting Behavior on the General Health of Office Workers." *J Lifestyle Med* 7(2): 69–75

Dragoo JL. 2013. "The effect of nonsteroidal anti-inflammatory drugs on tissue healing." *Knee Surg Sports Traumatol Arthrosc* 21(3):540–9

Dobrila-Dintinjana R, Nacinović-Duletić A. 2011. "Placebo in the treatment of pain." *Coll Antropol* 35 Suppl 2:319–23.

Ferrell C, Aspy C, Mold J. 2006. "Management of Prescription Refills in Primary Care: An Oklahoma Physicians Resource/Research Network (OKPRN) Study." *The Journal of the American Board of Family Medicine* 19(1):31–38

Frost H. 2004. "A 2003 Update of Bone Physiology and Wolff's Law for Clinicians." *Angle Orthod* 74:3–15

Garland E, et al. 2019. "Mindfulness-Oriented Recovery Enhancement remediates hedonic dysregulation in opioid users: Neural and affective evidence of target engagement." *Science Advances* 5(10): 1–12

Jain N, Himed K, Toth JM, Briley KC, Phillips FM, Khan SN. 2018. "Opioids delay healing of spinal fusion: a rabbit posterolateral lumbar fusion model. *Spine J.* 18(9):1659–1668

Jensen MC, Brant-Zawadzki MN, Obuchowski N, Modic MT, Malkasian D, Ross JS. 1994. "Magnetic resonance imaging of the lumbar spine in people without back pain." *N Engl J Med.* 331(2):69–73.

Khayambashi K, Ghoddosi N, Straub R, Powers C. 2015 "Hip Muscle Strength Predicts Noncontact Anterior Cruciate Ligament Injury in Male and Female Athletes: A Prospective Study." *Am J Sports Med* published online December 8, 2015

Kim Y, Wilkens LR, Schembre SM, Henderson BE, Kolonel LN, Goodman MT. 2013. "Insufficient and excessive amounts of sleep increase the risk of premature death from cardiovascular and other diseases: The Multiethnic Cohort Study." *Prev Med.* 57(4):377–85

Kumm J, Turkiewicz A, Zhang F, Englund M. 2018. "Structural abnormalities detected by knee magnetic resonance imaging are common in middle-aged subjects with and without risk factors for osteoarthritis." *Acta Orthop.* 89(5):535–540.

Lee D, et al. 2014. "Leisure-Time Running Reduces All-Cause and Cardiovascular Mortality Risk." *J Am Coll Cardiol.* 64(5): 472–481

Marras WS, Davis KG, Ferguson SA, Lucas BR, Gupta P. 2001. "Spine loading characteristics of patients with low back pain compared with asymptomatic individuals." Spine (Phila Pa 1976). 26(23):2566–74

Mosher TJ, Liu Y, Yang QX, Yao J, Smith R, Dardzinski BJ, Smith MB. 2004. "Age dependency of cartilage magnetic resonance imaging T2 relaxation times in asymptomatic women." *Arthritis Rheum.*50(9):2820–8.

Nakashima H, Yukawa Y, Suda K, Yamagata M, Ueta T, Kato F. 2015. "Abnormal findings on magnetic resonance images of the cervical spines in 1211 asymptomatic subjects." *Spine* (Phila Pa 1976) 40(6):392–8.

Rao VM, Levin DC, Parker L, Frangos AJ, Sunshine JH. 2011. "Trends in utilization rates of the various imaging modalities in emergency departments: nationwide Medicare data from 2000 to 2008." *J Am Coll Radiol.* 8(10):706–9.

Richards BL, et al. 2012. "The efficacy and safety of muscle relaxants in inflammatory arthritis: a Cochrane systematic review." J Rheumatol Suppl. 90:34–9.

Riera R. 2015. "Selective serotonin reuptake inhibitors for fibromyalgia syndrome." *Sao Paulo Med J.* 133(5):454

Rudd RA, Seth P, David F, Scholl L. 2016. "Increases in drug and opioid-involved overdose deaths—United States,

2010–2015." *Morbidity and Mortality Weekly Report.* 65:1445–1452

Schwartz L, Woloshin S. 2019. "Medical Marketing in the United States, 1997–2016." *JAMA.* 321(1):80–96.

Scully J. 2004. "What is a disease? *Disease, disability and their definitions."* *EMBO Rep* 5:650–653

Sihvonen R, et al. 2018. "Arthroscopic partial meniscectomy versus placebo surgery for a degenerative meniscus tear: a 2-year follow-up of the randomized controlled trial." *Ann Rheum Dis.* 77(2):188–195.

Smith MT, Haythornthwaite JA. 2004. "How do sleep disturbance and chronic pain inter-relate? Insights from the longitudinal and cognitive-behavioral clinical trials literature." *Sleep Med Rev.* 8(2):119–32. Review

Stecco A, et al. 2009. "Anatomical study of myofascial continuity in the anterior region of the upper limb." *J Bodyw Mov Ther.* 13(1):53–62.

Tozzi P. 2014. "Does fascia hold memories?" *J Bodyw Mov Ther.* 18:259-265

Vanini G. 2016. "Sleep Deprivation and Recovery Sleep Prior to a Noxious Inflammatory Insult." *Influence Characteristics and Duration of Pain Sleep.* 39(1): 133–142.

Violet TK. 2019. "Constructing the Gendered Risk of Illness in Lyrica Ads for Fibromyalgia: Fear of Isolation as a Motivating Narrative for Consumer Demand." *J Med Humanit.* Sep 2 epub.

Verrelst R, Van Tiggelen D, De Ridder R, Witvrouw E. 2018. "Decreased Average Power of the Hip External Muscles as a Predictive Parameter for Lower Extremity Injury in Women: A Prospective Study." *Clin J Sport Med.* 28(6):533–537

Wachholtz A, Gonzalez G. 2014. "Co-morbid pain and opioid addiction: long term effect of opioid maintenance on acute pain." *Drug Alcohol Depend.* 145:143–9.

Wilke J, Krause F, Vogt L, Banzer W. 2016. "What Is Evidence-Based About Myofascial Chains: A Systematic Review." *Arch Phys Med Rehabil.* 97(3):454–61

YaDeau JT, et al. 2016. "Duloxetine and Subacute Pain after Knee Arthroplasty when Added to a Multimodal Analgesic Regimen: A Randomized, Placebo-controlled, Triple-blinded Trial." *Anesthesiology.* 125(3):561–72

Yelin E, Weinstein S, King T. 2016. "The burden of musculoskeletal diseases in the United States." *Semin Arthritis Rheum.* 46(3):259–260.